Agora Health

Diabetes Defeated:

97 Most Powerful Secrets For Controlling Blood Sugar Levels Naturally

By Rachael Linkie
& Martin Hum PhD, DHD, Nutritional Therapist

CONTENTS

Introduction

How mainstream medicine is failing diabetes sufferers

Diabetes is fast turning into a serious problem. According to the charity Diabetes UK, there are approximately 2.9 million people diagnosed with diabetes. There are also thought to be around 850,000 people with undiagnosed diabetes.

Worse still, some experts are now predicting that these figures are set to more than double over the next 10 years. This is extremely worrying considering that the condition causes more deaths than breast and prostate cancer combined. There has also been a huge growth in complication rates. Diabetes is now the biggest single cause of amputation, stroke, blindness, and end-stage kidney failure.

Perhaps most shocking of all is the poor level of diabetes care. Diabetes is a serious and complex condition, that's all-too-often misunderstood, even by most doctors. In a recent report, Diabetes UK points out that the NHS is falling woefully short of the vision it set itself in 2001, for diabetes services to be delivered by 2013 (*State of the Nation 2012: England. Diabetes UK. May 2012*). The report says that diabetes prevention and management have not been successfully tackled, meaning that diabetes continues to increase, along with its associated complications and costs.

In fact, a report just out from the Public Accounts Committee – a group of MPs whose job is to report on how efficiently and effectively public resources are used – reveals that many diabetics are being badly let down by the NHS. It estimates that 24,000 people die prematurely every year because their diabetes has not been managed effectively, with many more developing avoidable complications, such as blindness and kidney disease (*Public Accounts Committee – Seventeenth Report. Department of Health: The management of adult diabetes services in the NHS. House of Commons, October 2012*).

There seems to be something of a postcode lottery when it comes to diabetes. Diabetes UK claims there is wide variability across the country, which means that there are still significant numbers of people with diabetes who do not have access to the standards of care they need and deserve. There has to be more accurate, early diagnosis, more effective treatment and better adherence to the standards regarding laboratory tests.

Doctors have plenty of guidance on the checks that should be made on each person with diabetes, and yet the report reveals that two-thirds of adults with type 1 diabetes and half of people with type 2 diabetes fail to get the annual tests and investigations that they should. For children, the figures are scandalously worse. In England, an incredible 96 per cent of children don't receive all of the annual routine health checks. That is simply shameful and increases the risk that potentially life-threatening, diabetes-related complications will not be picked up on at an early stage.

Even if you are getting the tests you need, don't assume that the treatment you are prescribed will put things right. On average, in England, only 63 per cent of diabetics undergoing treatment have blood sugar (glycosylated haemoglobin, HbA1c) within the recommended level. For blood pressure and cholesterol, these averages drop to 51 per cent and 40 per cent respectively. The report sums up the standard of diabetes care in England as "too little, too late, too variable".

Drugs are all-too-often the first line of treatment

Doctors routinely prescribe medication following a diabetes diagnosis... and this can put you on the path to a lifetime's dependence on drugs. Both type 1 and type 2 diabetics may need to inject themselves with insulin every day and there is also a range of diabetic medications that vary in their effectiveness and side effects. At worst, these medications have been linked with heart attacks, pancreatic cancer, bladder cancer, stroke, osteoporosis and vision loss.

In some cases medication is vital but in others the condition can be successfully managed without drugs. As you're about to discover in this report, diabetes, especially in its early stages, can be controlled and even fully reversed in some cases through lifestyle changes such as diet, exercise and supplements.

While dietary advice is given by many doctors, it's normally the wrong advice... with many doctors and dieticians still advocating a low fat, high carbohydrate diet, which is guaranteed to elevate a diabetic's blood sugar levels further and encourage weight gain. In addition to receiving misguided dietary advice, diabetics often walk away from their doctor's surgery armed with brochures, almost all of which are published by pharmaceutical companies, which emphasise the importance of medication...

How the drug companies have turned diabetes into a highly profitable 'cash cow'

The bottom line: As long as diabetics need drugs, Big Pharma makes billions. The number of prescriptions written for such drugs rocketed to an unbelievable £40 million last year, up 50 per cent in just five years, a trend that threatens to bankrupt the NHS if it continues (*Prescribing for Diabetes in England: 2005/6 to 2011/12. The Health and Social Care Information Centre. 14 August 2012. http://www.ic.nhs.uk/webfiles/publications/007_Primary_Care/Prescribing/diabetes20056to201112/Prescribing_for_Diabetes_in_England_20056_to_201112.pdf*). To put it another way, every taxpayer in England donates roughly £50 a year to the pharmaceutical industry, for diabetes drugs alone.

Danish drugs maker Novo Nordisk says its net profit grew by 29 per cent in the second quarter of 2012, to £570 million, chiefly spurred by strong sales of its new diabetes drugs. US drugs giant Merck reported first-quarter profits in 2012 that exceeded all expectations, due to higher sales of its diabetes treatments, with net income rising by a staggering 67 per cent to £1.1 billion.

3

Profits are all-too-often put before safety

A recent report accuses the pharmaceutical industry of putting profits before patients, by being too focused on marketing and not devoting enough resources to developing new, breakthrough treatments. This was not the conclusion of some anti-capitalist agitators, but of two distinguished University professors, writing in the *British Medical Journal* (*BMJ 2012; 345: e4348*). In their report, they point out that while research and development costs rose by £21.7 billion between 1995 and 2010, revenues increased six times faster – by £127 billion.

The biggest profits, it seems, come not from developing genuinely new drugs, but from tinkering with or combining existing ones and then marketing the resulting product aggressively, irrespective of its real effectiveness and with scant regard to its safety. Independent reviews suggest, incredibly, that 85 to 90 per cent of new drugs provide little benefit over existing treatments.

In fact, the last thing the drug companies want is to find a cure for diabetes. The big money comes from finding something that reduces the symptoms but allows the underlying disease process to continue, leading to more and more prescriptions being written.

The dirty dealings and cover ups of the drugs industry

In July, GlaxoSmithKline (GSK), agreed to pay a $3 billion fine and plead guilty to a felony in the US, in connection with the marketing of its diabetes drug Avandia (rosiglitazone). GSK admitted that, from 2001 to 2007, it hid data about Avandia's risks of heart attack and congestive heart failure.

According to the US Food and Drug Administration (FDA), Avandia could have caused up to 100,000 heart attacks. More than 50,000 individual lawsuits have been filed in state and federal courts across the US, citing GSK's failure to inform patients about the potentially life-threatening side effects, including heart attack, stroke, heart failure, bone fractures, vision loss, and death, that have been linked to the drug. GSK's biggest rival, Takeda Pharmaceutical Co, which makes a similar diabetes drug called Actos (pioglitazone), have also been accused of withholding safety data, because they wanted to make it appear safer than Avandia. Actos' side effects include bladder cancer and congestive heart failure.

Here in the UK, things may not be much better. The European Medicines Agency (EMA), which licenses drugs in the UK and Europe, keeps much of the data about their safety and efficacy secret. Almost 30 per cent of new drugs approved by the EMA have received safety warnings within 10 years of being put on the market.

The bitter truth is that pharmaceutical companies are not researching diligently to develop ever safer and more effective drugs that will improve the quality of people's lives. They are looking instead to create a smokescreen of glossy advertising and to make as much money as possible before their products are discovered to be worthless or even dangerous.

However, there are plenty of things you can do to reduce your reliance on these potentially-harmful drugs...

Discover how to fight back against diabetes

As already mentioned, it is possible to reverse diabetes, especially in its early stages, through diet and exercise, and reduce, and in some cases even eliminate, the need to take insulin. However, it's important to point out that every person's diabetes is different and you should never stop taking any medication without discussing your own situation with your doctor.

Making the simple changes outlined in this report can also lead to other improvements – from reversing fatigue and boosting your energy levels to reducing your blood pressure and triglyceride (blood fat) levels, which in turn helps lower your risk of a heart attack or stroke. By following the advice given you'll also lose any excess weight, which in itself brings considerable improvements in blood glucose regulation; and, for some people, return to a healthy weight brings complete remission of their diabetes.

The real diabetes truth

This report aims to shatter common myths about the condition, and will tell you what really works for sufferers, based on cutting-edge research. One of the most promising areas of research involves the use of specific nutritional supplements and herbal remedies to ward off diabetes. In the coming pages, you're about to discover the best of these natural breakthroughs and safe alternatives that can help bring your blood sugar levels down and transform your health in the process.

After reading about the impressive results they're getting in clinical trials and learning about the extraordinary case studies of diabetics whose lives they've helped turn around, you'll no doubt wonder why this important information is not more widely known and why your doctor hasn't told you about it. Well, the fact is there is no money to be made from vitamins and other natural remedies, so as a result the drug companies prefer to promote their expensive, synthetic products instead (irrespective of whether they work or not). And most doctors rely on the drug companies for their treatment information.

While it's extremely important to work closely with your doctor and have your blood sugar levels regularly monitored, it's also important to be well informed and make sure you are getting all the necessary checks... including those that can pick up on any complications before they reach crisis point.

Rather than waste precious time trying to trawl through all the available information on the best diabetes preventatives and breakthroughs out there, we've done the hard work for you. With *Diabetes Defeated: 97 Most Powerful Secrets For Controlling Blood Sugar Levels Naturally* at your fingertips you'll have access to easy-to-follow, practical advice and potentially life-saving information. Armed with this knowledge you can expect to feel empowered and confident that you can work alongside your doctor to make informed decisions about your health and about what treatment approach gives you the best chance of successfully managing your diabetes (or even possibly reversing it).

At the end of this report you'll find a comprehensive list of further resources to turn to, including reliable books and websites on the condition, and contact details of diabetes' organisations and support networks.

Chapter 1

What is diabetes?

Diabetes causes blood sugar levels to become damagingly high because the hormone insulin, which is produced by the pancreas, is not regulating it properly. In a healthy person insulin lowers blood sugar by signalling the body's cells to absorb glucose from the bloodstream where it is converted into energy. Diabetes mellitus ('sugar diabetes') – which differs from diabetes insipidus (a rare disorder of the pituitary gland, which has similar symptoms to diabetes mellitus, but without disturbances in sugar metabolism) – is divided into three main types: Type 1 diabetes, type 2 diabetes and gestational diabetes:

1. Type 1 diabetes, once known as juvenile diabetes or insulin-dependent diabetes, usually becomes apparent in childhood or adolescence. It is an auto-immune condition in which the body's immune system destroys the insulin-producing cells (known as beta cells) of the pancreas, resulting in little or no insulin being produced. Without insulin, blood sugar cannot enter the cells and instead stays in the bloodstream where levels become dangerously high, which in turn can cause serious damage to all organ systems in the body.

It isn't clear why the body's immune system turns on the beta cells, but a number of explanations and possible triggers have been proposed. These include infection with a specific virus or bacteria, exposure to food-borne chemical toxins, exposure as a very young infant to cow's milk, where an as yet unidentified component triggers the autoimmune reaction. As with other autoimmune diseases, an underlying genetic disposition seems to play a part, leaving some people more vulnerable to these triggers. In rare cases, damage to the pancreas by tumours, toxins or injury (including surgery), can also lead to type 1 diabetes.

In type 1 diabetes, symptoms tend to develop rapidly over a couple of weeks. Common symptoms include increased thirst, a frequent need to pass urine (especially at night), tiredness and fatigue, genital itching or recurrent thrush.

In most cases, blood sugar levels are managed through daily injections of insulin and, sometimes, other medicines. Some type 1 diabetics don't require insulin injections – they may be able to get by on a minimum of insulin if they have a few functioning beta cells (namely new ones are produced as soon as others are destroyed).

2. Type 2 diabetes, once referred to as adult-onset diabetes and non-insulin-dependent diabetes mellitus (NIDDM), is the most common form of diabetes. In the UK, about 90 per cent of all adults with diabetes have type 2. It is a metabolic condition that can be diagnosed at any age and is often preceded by metabolic syndrome (also known as syndrome X) – a collection of risk factors including excessive abdominal fat, elevated triglyceride and CRP levels, low HDL (the 'good' form of cholesterol), high blood pressure, and a fasting glucose level that would indicate possible insulin resistance. Three or more of these symptoms are all that's required to diagnose metabolic syndrome... which, in addition to putting you at greater risk of diabetes, also increases your odds of developing heart disease.

Whereas type 2 diabetes was once seen only in the over-40s, it is now being diagnosed in a growing number of younger people and even children. It is frightening to think that our increasingly unhealthy lifestyles, which have increased the numbers of people (including children) who are overweight and obese, has led to a huge rise in the number of type 2 diabetics. In fact, 80 per cent of diabetics are overweight – waist circumference is particularly important: a waist size greater than 35in in women and 40in in men has recently been shown to significantly increase the risk of developing diabetes, high blood pressure and heart disease.

However, it's important to bear in mind that around 20 per cent of people diagnosed with type 2 diabetes are normal weight or underweight. In addition to weight, other factors that can cause type 2 diabetes include a sedentary lifestyle; ageing (over 40s are more at risk); or those over 25 and

African-Caribbean, Asian or from a minority ethnic group; a family history of diabetes (children of people with type 2 diabetes have a one in three chance of developing the condition themselves); being a woman who has given birth to a large baby; smoking; certain medicines; and any illness or disease that damages the pancreas and affects its ability to produce insulin, such as pancreatitis.

Type 2 diabetes occurs when the pancreas does not produce enough insulin to control your blood glucose level, or the body's cells do not react to insulin. The latter is known as insulin resistance, which is how the condition usually begins... the body's cells become unable to use insulin properly, as the specific insulin receptors on the cells stop reacting. Sugar instead stays in the blood and causes trouble. Over time, the type 2 diabetic's cells become less and less sensitive to insulin. This puts pressure on the pancreas to release huge amounts of insulin to try to force the cells to react.

One of insulin's roles is to reduce fat metabolism while simultaneously promoting fat storage. While muscle cells become insulin resistant, fat cells do not, meaning that sugar is absorbed into fat cells as they have nowhere else to go. The result is that these fat cells get bigger, which is why many diabetics are obese. Eventually the pancreas becomes 'exhausted' as a result of having to produce so much insulin and loses this ability.

New hope for restoring insulin production in type 2 diabetes

Until now, the assumption has been that the pancreas stops producing insulin because the beta-cells, the specific cells in the pancreas that secrete this hormone, have died. New research has shown, however, that these vital cells have not been killed off but have simply reverted to a neutral (undifferentiated) state. In other words, they are no longer receiving the genetic information that tells them what their job is in the body.

The new study was carried out using specially-bred mice, at Columbia

University Medical Centre in the United States (*Cell. 2012; 150 (6): 1223*). It showed that a protein called FOXO1 is central to the function of pancreatic beta-cells and to their 'disappearance' in type 2 diabetes. FOXO1 is a transcription factor, a protein that controls when genes are switched on or off. It is part of a set of pancreatic transcription factors that regulate every aspect of the development and functioning of the pancreas.

The researchers discovered that FOXO1 is necessary to maintain the identity of beta cells. Under the metabolic stress of insulin resistance, beta cells gradually become depleted in FOXO1 and start to change into a neutral state, in which they are no longer capable of producing insulin, probably as a self-protective mechanism.

As Professor Domenico Accili, who led the research, explained: "Currently, we give patients medications that force beta cells to work even harder. But it's like flogging a dying horse. You can push beta cells only so far. Our findings would suggest that treatment should begin by giving beta cells a rest, by administering insulin." This exciting new research opens up the possibility that the process is reversible and that beta-cells could be given back their identity and function by re-establishing the activity of FOXO1.

Why insulin-promoting medications are best avoided

As Professor Accili states, it's true that medications that aim to make a failing pancreas produce more insulin are a waste of time. Much worse than that, they could increase your risks of pancreatitis (severe, life-threatening inflammation of the pancreas) and pancreatic cancer, according to recent research (*Gastroenterology. 2011; 141 (1): 150–156*). Even the most common side effects of digestive upsets, nausea, faintness, tremor and weight gain are best avoided.

Giving the pancreas a rest is also essential. However, Professor Accili's view that administering insulin is the best way to do this is questionable.

In certain cases, insulin may be medically essential, but in many cases type 2 diabetics can control their blood sugar levels perfectly well by following a low glycaemic load diet and the other measures outlined in *Diabetes Defeated: 97 Most Powerful Secrets For Controlling Blood Sugar Levels Naturally.*

The unnecessary administration of insulin, leading to an excess of the hormone in your system, pushes up your cholesterol level and blood pressure, damages your arteries and promotes weight gain. People who inject insulin also have a significantly higher risk of cancer, although the reason for this is unclear.

Certain herbal remedies could have the ability to coax beta-cells out of the neutral state they have reverted to and get them producing insulin again. Further research is needed to reveal the mechanisms involved, but the initial signs are encouraging.

Gymnema, fenugreek and *Pterocarpus marsupium* are herbs that have been used for centuries in India as traditional remedies for diabetes. An extract of gymnema has been found to significantly regenerate beta-cells in diabetic rats (*Phytomedicine. 2010; 17 (13): 1033-1039*). Fenugreek contains an amino acid called 4-hydroxyisoleucine, which may stimulate the secretion of insulin. In animal studies, fenugreek oil not only increased insulin production but also protected beta-cells from oxidative damage (*Immunopharmacol Immunotoxicol. 2010; 32 (3): 437-445*).

An extract of the bark of the Indian Kino Tree, *Pterocarpus marsupium*, has been shown to have a regenerative effect on the pancreatic beta cells (India *J Pharmacol. 1980; 12: 123-127*). In animal experiments, an extract of the hardwood had potent antidiabetic effects, by both stimulating insulin production and acting in the same way as insulin in allowing glucose to enter muscle cells (*J Ethnopharmacol. 2012; 141 (1): 72-79*).

Type 2 diabetes symptoms are similar to those of type 1 diabetes

While the symptoms between these two types of diabetes are similar, type 2 diabetes symptoms typically develop more slowly and are usually milder than those of type 1 diabetes. They include fatigue, frequent hunger, excessive thirst and a frequent need to urinate. The condition can also cause blurred vision, constipation, weight loss and loss of muscle bulk, genital itching and regular bouts of thrush, a dry mouth and dry or itchy skin. It is important to see your doctor immediately if you suspect you may be developing diabetes, as it can be a life-threatening condition.

However, the condition doesn't always cause symptoms and they're not always severe in those that do experience them, which is why it is sometimes referred to as the 'silent assassin'. In fact, type 2 diabetes can remain undetected for 10 years or more, which may account for why 50 per cent of people show signs of complications when they are eventually diagnosed.

Research into the causes of diabetes is on-going, and there is now evidence to suggest that...

• Chronic inflammation can cause type 2 diabetes

While insulin resistance is a feature of type 2 diabetes and is generally thought of as a precursor to the disease, the fact remains that only about a third of people with insulin resistance go on to develop type 2 diabetes involving impaired insulin production. So what makes these people different? Genetic factors, as well as environmental ones like diet and exercise doubtless play a major part, but chronic inflammation is also involved.

Recently, a German study showed that people infected with cytomegalovirus (CMV), which is usually carried without any ill effects, are at greater risk of developing type 2 diabetes in later life (*Immun Ageing. 2012 Aug 28;9(1):18. [Epub ahead of print]*). The researchers investigated glucose regulation and the presence of antibodies to CMV in elderly people.

They found that those people who had CMV antibodies had higher blood sugar readings than those without the antibodies and that 17.2 per cent of subjects with CMV antibodies had diabetes, compared to 7.9 per cent of those without.

If you become infected with CMV, you carry it for life. Although it is normally dormant and produces no symptoms, it can become active at any point in time, provoking a reaction from the immune system that involves inflammation in many body organs and tissues, but often most noticeably in the salivary glands under the jawbone. The German researchers suggest that CMV could either directly affect insulin production by damaging the pancreatic beta-cells or act indirectly by causing the immune system to attack the pancreas.

Other new research from Denmark has found that patients with the skin disease psoriasis are also at higher than average risk of developing type 2 diabetes. The results of a 13-year study involving over four million people, including 50,000 patients with psoriasis, were presented to the European Society of Cardiology Congress in Munich, Germany, in August (*European Society of Cardiology Congress 2012, Munich, Germany, Aug. 25-29, 2012*). The data showed a rate of 3.6 new cases of diabetes per 1,000 people per year in those without psoriasis, which rose to 6.9 in people with mild psoriasis and 9.7 in those with the severe form of the disease.

Psoriasis is not caused by an infection. It is an autoimmune disease, in which the immune system attacks the skin cells, and it affects approximately 125 million people worldwide. It is characterised by chronic inflammation, which the Danish researchers believe may explain the increased risk of both diabetes and cardiovascular problems seen in patients with the disease.

Don't risk the side effects caused by anti-inflammatory drugs

What these two studies have in common is the link between chronic inflammation and an increased risk of type 2 diabetes. Inflammation is a natural and necessary part of the immune system's defence mechanism and is beneficial when it is a temporary and local response to a threat to the body. However, when inflammation becomes unregulated and persists as an on-going condition, it can seriously disrupt the body's vital processes and is a factor in most chronic diseases.

One of the adverse effects of chronic inflammation is the destruction of the insulin-producing beta-cells in the pancreas, which causes type 1 diabetes when it involves an auto-immune condition and type 2 diabetes when it results from metabolic imbalance.

Although your doctor has an arsenal of anti-inflammatory drugs at his or her disposal, these come with a long list of side effects that you would do better to avoid. At the top of this list come painful peptic ulcers and internal bleeding. Non-steroidal anti-inflammatories (NSAIDs) have also been associated with an increased risk of heart attack and stroke and commonly cause nausea, vomiting, heartburn, dizziness, constipation, diarrhoea, increased blood pressure and erectile dysfunction.

There are plenty of safer alternatives. As usual, this isn't rocket science!

Follow these tips to control inflammation naturally

- Cut down the omega-6 fatty acids in your diet, which come from oils such as corn, sunflower, safflower and peanut. These are the raw materials from which inflammatory chemicals are produced. Take a fish oil supplement to increase the ratio of omega-3 to omega-6 fatty acids.

- If you are overweight, do your best to lose the extra pounds by following a low glycaemic load (low-GL) diet. Body fat is a factory for inflammatory compounds.

- Take a supplement of curcumin (the active ingredient in the spice turmeric). This is one of the most diverse and powerful natural anti-inflammatory agents known and out-performs several anti-inflammatory drugs, without the side effects. It is one of the key ingredients in Solgar's Cherry Turmeric Complex (see page 183 for more details).

- Support your immune system, so that it does not malfunction. In recent years, the importance of beta-glucans for immune function has become well established. Take a good quality beta-glucan supplement, such as Bio-Glucan Plus.

• Environmental toxins: The hidden culprit behind diabetes

Earlier this year, a Korean study showed that toxic chemicals in the environment may be making us both more obese and more diabetic (*Epidemiol Health. 2012; 34:e2012002*). The researchers found that blood levels of chemicals classed as 'persistent organic pollutants', or POPs, such as organochlorine pesticides and polychlorinated biphenyls (PCBs), were strongly and consistently linked to type 2 diabetes and to obesity, insulin resistance and unhealthy blood fat profiles. The prevalence of diabetes was five times higher in people with the greatest concentrations of toxins than in those with the least.

The real bombshell in this research, though, was the finding that in people with low levels of POPs obesity is not linked to diabetes. The link only becomes apparent when levels of pollutants are 'moderate' or 'high'. The implication is that virtually all of the diabetes risk that comes with obesity is attributable to environmental toxins and that obesity is only a vehicle for such chemicals. The strong link between diabetes and obesity (sometimes referred to as 'diabesity') is only a reality because of the environmental poisons that we carry inside us.

The toxic burden in our air, food and water – and so in our bodies – grows higher year by year. Around three billion tonnes of artificial chemicals are manufactured worldwide every year. Some of these we expose ourselves to in the form of toiletries and domestic products, such as detergents and air fresheners. For instance, women have higher levels of toxins called phthalates than do men, due to their greater use of personal grooming products. New research from Harvard Medical School has shown that having a high level of phthalates could double your chances of developing type 2 diabetes (*Environ Health Perspect. 2012; 120(9):1307-1313*).

Other toxins come from the air we breathe and from our drinking water. Much of the burden, though, is passed on to us when we eat the meat (and particularly the fat) of animals. Agricultural chemicals present in animal feeds and on pastures accumulate in animal fat. So do toxins that are circulated around the globe in the oceans. The incidence of diabetes is five times higher in native people in the Canadian Arctic than in the general population, as a result of the environmental pollutants that accumulate in their traditional diet of wild game and fish (*Int J Circumpolar Health. 2009; 68(4):316-326*).

According to a recent review article in *Alternative Therapies in Health and Medicine* (*Altern Ther Health Med. 2010; 16(2):56-58*), toxins slow down the metabolism and contribute to weight gain and diabetes. They act through multiple mechanisms, which include disrupting enzymes, impairing glucose transport, causing oxidative stress, inducing inflammatory cytokines, and damaging the energy-producing mitochondria inside cells. Toxins induce insulin resistance by interfering with the function of a class of transcription factors (proteins that switch on genes) called PPARs, which are needed for optimal insulin function, blood sugar control and the regulation of inflammation.

How to protect yourself from environmental toxins

None of us can avoid environmental pollutants entirely, but it is prudent to take the following steps to ensure that your toxic burden is as low as possible:

- Don't use more household chemicals and personal grooming

products than absolutely necessary. Take a look at less dangerous alternatives (The Green People: www.greenpeople.co.uk manufacture a range of skin care, hair care and cosmetic products that don't use any harsh chemicals and select only the finest natural and organic ingredients. In addition they use fair trade ingredients that have not been tested on animals. They also produce chemical-free products for babies.

- Opt for organic foods (organic meat in particular) and avoid cured or processed meat products.

- Improve liver and bowel functions by including fresh vegetable juices and healthy amounts of fibre, probiotics, and digestive enzymes every day.

- Help your liver to break down and remove toxins, by getting plenty of sleep and by taking supplements of milk thistle, n-acetyl cysteine, and alpha lipoic acid.

- Do a one-week 'detox', twice a year. Talk to a nutritional therapist for advice on how to do this.

- If your health allows, work up a sweat regularly from vigorous exercise or by taking a sauna.

- **Could *Helicobacter pylori* bacteria be responsible for your blood sugar problems?**

You may have heard of *Helicobacter pylori* (usually shortened to *H. pylori*), the bacterium that is responsible for causing stomach ulcers. Around half of the world's population is estimated to carry *H. pylori*, but 80 per cent of people who have it suffer no symptoms. When it does cause problems, abdominal pain and nausea are common, with peptic ulcers developing in 10 to 20 per cent of people harbouring the bug. *H. pylori* is usually acquired before the age of ten and lives in the mucous layer lining the stomach, where it persists for decades.

A new study by researchers in New York has discovered that stomach problems are not the only way in which *H. pylori* can damage our health (*J Infect Dis. 2012; 205(8):1195-1202*). Its presence has now been linked to elevated levels of glycosylated haemoglobin (HbA1c), an important marker for blood glucose levels and diabetes. This association was found to be even stronger in obese and overweight individuals.

Scientists have long suspected that there may be a link between *H. pylori* and diabetes. In 1996, a Dutch study reported a higher incidence of antibodies to the bacterium in diabetic patients than in non-diabetic controls (*Dig Dis Sci. 1996; 41(3):458-461*). A literature review carried out last year in Greece also linked *H. pylori* with insulin resistance (*Helicobacter. 2011; 16(2):79-88*).

What makes the new study different is that for the first time *H. pylori* infection has been shown to affect the blood level of glycosylated haemoglobin, a standard test measurement that indicates an on-going problem with high blood sugar. It is also the first study to analyse data from two large, independent samples of the general population, which makes its results more reliable. Previous studies have mostly looked at small groups of patients, usually in a hospital setting.

The researchers who carried out the latest study believe that the bacterium may affect the levels of two important digestive hormones, ghrelin and leptin, which help regulate blood glucose, leading to elevated blood sugar and, in the longer term, to higher levels of glycosylated haemoglobin. Ghrelin, sometimes called the 'hunger hormone', decreases calorie-burning and promotes weight gain. Leptin reduces appetite and boosts calorie-burning. Previous research has linked *H. pylori* with changes in the levels of these hormones (*J Clin Endocrinol Metab. 2008; 93(6):2350-2357*).

This research suggests that, in theory, testing for and eradicating *H.*

pylori might protect overweight adults from developing diabetes. But it is not yet clear whether people who already have diabetes would actually benefit from antibiotic treatment. In a clinical trial in Japan, *H. pylori* infections were eradicated in patients with type 2 diabetes who had no peptic ulcers or other complications. Surprisingly, no change was seen in their glycosylated haemoglobin levels as a result of the treatment and the patients tended to put on weight in the months following the eradication (*Hepatogastroenterology. 2012; 59 (114)*).

For the time being, while it is worth discussing this research with your doctor, it seems that there is no generally accepted protocol for *H. pylori* eradication treatment in the absence of gastritis or stomach ulcer symptoms. In the meantime, follow a low carbohydrate diet, particularly one that is low in wheat products, since wheat gluten tends to irritate the gut and favours the growth of *H. pylori*. Eating plenty of berry fruits and garlic and taking supplements of fish oils, lactobacillus and blackcurrant seed oil have also been found to help in the eradication of the bacterium.

• New evidence shows that statin drugs can cause diabetes

It is well established that heart attacks and strokes are the major cause of death in diabetes sufferers, which is why many doctors tend to prescribe statin drugs to such patients in an attempt to reduce the risk. Statins are a class of drugs that reduce levels of cholesterol, an essential substance in the body that has become the scapegoat for the growing problem of cardiovascular disease.

Now, though, the US Food and Drug Administration (FDA) has issued new labelling guidelines for statin drugs, warning users that taking them can result in elevated blood sugar levels, diabetes and memory loss. This is in addition to their previously known side effects of muscle damage and liver disease.

The first signs of a link with diabetes were evident as long ago as 2004, with a research report that statin drugs disrupt insulin signalling, the process through which insulin moves glucose from the bloodstream into muscle and fat cells (*J Biol Chem. 2004; 279 (37): 38353-9*). The implications of this study appear to have been ignored, however, until two recent meta-analyses took a hard look at the link between statins and diabetes.

The first of these, published in June 2011, involved 33,000 patients enrolled in five major clinical trials using statins. It concluded that, overall, statin use caused around one additional case of diabetes for every 500 patients treated and the higher the dose, the higher the risk (*JAMA. 2011; 305 (24): 2556-2564*). This figure is a bit misleading, though, since it includes earlier trials of the weaker statin drugs. The more potent versions being prescribed today are likely to be linked to a much bigger diabetes problem, especially at higher doses.

Statins block an essential metabolic pathway

The second meta-analysis, the results of which were published in January 2012, looked at data from almost 154,000 postmenopausal women (*Arch Intern Med. 2012; 172 (2): 144-152*). It revealed that women taking statins had a 48 per cent greater risk of diabetes, compared with similar women not taking statins. These findings are not just chance occurrences. By blocking the production of cholesterol in the liver, statin drugs also block the production of a related substance called dolichol, which plays an important role in sugar metabolism and insulin sensitivity. Incidentally, dolichol levels have been found to be unusually low in people with Alzheimer's disease, which could go some way towards explaining why statin use has also been linked with memory loss.

So, what do you do if you are currently taking statins? Before anything else, talk to your doctor about these findings. Don't be fobbed off with assurances that this is a minor side effect that is outweighed by the benefits of taking statins. A 2011 Cochrane Review showed, basically, that taking statins does almost nothing to reduce heart attack risk in people who have not previously experienced a heart attack (*Cochrane Database Syst Rev. 2011; (1): CD004816*).

If you already have diabetes, your cholesterol level is not likely to be an additional risk factor. And don't let your doctor persuade you that statins will reduce your likelihood of peripheral neuropathy (nerve damage) as a complication of diabetes, either. A 2002 population study estimated the risks of neuropathy in statin users and concluded that long term exposure to these drugs significantly increased the risk (*Neurology. 2002; 58 (9): 1333-7*).

While drugs may play a useful role in some situations, for the vast majority of us, whether or not we have been diagnosed as having diabetes, eating healthily and getting enough exercise remain our best front line defence against heart disease.

- ## It's not just statins... these prescription drugs could be a major cause of diabetes too

We all know that prescription drugs come with a variety of side effects in some people. Things like tummy upsets, constipation, headaches, drowsiness, dizziness and nausea are fairly common. What most of us don't think about when handed a prescription by our doctor is that the medicine could set us on the path towards metabolic syndrome and type 2 diabetes. Yet, that is the shocking truth – not for some rarely prescribed drug for a condition you've never heard of, but for whole classes of commonly prescribed medications that together make up the vast majority of prescriptions written in the UK.

Steroids: A class of frequently prescribed steroid drugs called glucocorticoids (such as prednisolone) is also known to affect blood sugar control and lead to type 2 diabetes. The medical community is well aware of 'steroid diabetes' as a condition that arises in people who have to take these drugs for an extended period, such as kidney transplant patients. But if your GP prescribes you a glucocorticoid for your asthma, eczema or irritable bowel syndrome, you may not be warned of this risk. Glucocorticoids raise blood sugar levels by promoting insulin resistance in the liver and muscle cells. At higher doses, they also impair the function of insulin-producing beta cells in the pancreas, reducing the release of insulin (*Metabolism. 2012*

Nov 16 [Epub ahead of print]).

Beta-blockers: Another mainstay of drug-based medicine, beta blockers are used to treat a wide variety of conditions, including high blood pressure, angina, abnormal heart rhythm, overactive thyroid, glaucoma, anxiety and migraine. These drugs not only increase blood sugar levels in those who don't have diabetes, but may worsen blood sugar control in people with diabetes and also blunt the warning symptoms when hypoglycaemia occurs (*Heart Fail Clin. 2012; 8 (4): xiii-xvi*). A massive study involving nearly 20,000 patients established a clear connection between the use of older beta-blocker drugs, such as atenolol, and type 2 diabetes (*Diabetes Care. 2008; 31 (5): 982-988*).

Antidepressants: Several studies have linked the long-term use of antidepressants, one of the most frequently prescribed kinds of medication in the UK, with a raised risk of type 2 diabetes. All types of antidepressants, including tricyclic and SSRIs, are implicated. A recent major study, which examined the health data of more than 168,000 people, concluded that, even after adjusting for weight gain (a common side effect of antidepressants), people taking these drugs had an elevated risk of type 2 diabetes (*Diabetologia. 2012; 55 (1): 63-72*).

The list goes on and on...

Other classes of drugs have also been linked with raised blood sugar levels, metabolic syndrome or type 2 diabetes. They include:

* **Blood pressure drugs**. A long-term study found that they were associated with new onset diabetes in 20 per cent of patients who took them and with a consequent increased risk of heart attack and stroke in these patients (*J Hypertens. 2007; 25(6): 1311-7*).

* **Diuretics**, particularly the thiazide type, which reduce blood potassium levels and interfere with the release of insulin by the pancreas (*Hypertension. 2010; 55 (1): 15-17*).

- **Mood stabilisers,** such as clozapine, quetiapine and risperidone, which have been found to cause metabolic syndrome, including raised blood sugar and blood fat levels, abdominal obesity and high blood pressure (*J Exp Clin Med.2012; 4 (2): 103–107*).

- **Anti-epilepsy drug** sodium valproate (Epilim), which is often also prescribed for bipolar disorder and can interfere with the mechanism by which cells take up glucose, leading to raised blood sugar levels (*J Cell Biochem.2005; 96 (4): 775-785*).

If you already have diabetes or metabolic syndrome, it is vital that you are aware of the damage that the drugs mentioned above could do to your blood sugar control. Ask your doctor how any medications you are taking could affect your glucose metabolism. Sometimes it is a case of weighing one risk against another, but often there are safer drugs or non-drug alternatives that can be just as effective. Just don't stop any medication without letting your doctor know.

• Autism linked to diabetes and insulin levels

In 2011 a review of the genetic and biochemical abnormalities associated with autistic spectrum disorder (ASD) revealed a possible link between this neurological condition and type 2 diabetes (*Frontiers in Endocrinology, 2011; 2 DOI: 10.3389/fendo.2011.00054*). Dr Michael Stern, who led the research at Rice University in Houston, Texas, believes that both these health problems share a common underlying cause – impaired glucose tolerance and too much insulin in the bloodstream.

Doctors have suspected for years that there may be a link between ASD and gestational diabetes, in which pregnant women temporarily develop high blood sugar levels. However, several reviews of ASD risk factors have failed to make a clear statistical connection or identify a mechanism to explain this observation.

In May 2012, a study reported that obese mothers were 67 per cent more likely to have an autistic child than normal-weight mothers and that mothers with diabetes were also 67 per cent more likely to have a child with developmental delays (*Pediatrics. 2012; 129 (5): e1121-1128*). Even children without ASD born to diabetic mothers had problems with socialisation and language, when compared with the non-ASD children of healthy women.

So, how does a mother's high insulin level cause a neurological problem in her unborn child? Dr Stern believes that he finally has the answer. At least four genes associated with an increased frequency of autism are known to produce proteins that play key roles in a biochemical pathway known as PI3K/Tor. It turns out that this is the major pathway for insulin signals within cells, through which insulin does its job of moving glucose from the bloodstream into the cells. And it appears that insulin can affect nerve synapses in the brain in a remarkably similar way to the defects associated with autism.

This strongly suggests that high insulin levels, whether due to type 1 or 2 diabetes or to gestational diabetes, could affect the synapses in the developing foetus in a way that causes damage typical of ASD. A pilot study in Greece has given the parents of children with ASD some hope that a low carbohydrate diet may help them. When 18 children aged between four and ten, with autistic behaviour, followed an Atkins-like, low carbohydrate diet for six months, they all showed improvements in their condition: significant in two children, moderate in eight and slight in the remaining eight (*J Child Neurol. 2003; 18 (2): 113-118*).

Of course, ASD is a complex disorder and several other factors are likely to be involved in its initiation and progress. But what these studies show is that insulin is not just an issue for people with diabetes, it can have widespread effects in the body and the brain. And low carbohydrate diets can help resolve health problems other than diabetes, metabolic syndrome and obesity.

3. Gestational diabetes occurs in between five and ten per cent of pregnant women, during the last three months of pregnancy. The incidence of gestational diabetes has risen considerably in recent years, in line with that of type 2 diabetes (*Diabetes Care. 2007; 30 Suppl 2:S141-146*). Two main factors are thought to be behind this condition – hormones produced in the placenta causing insulin resistance and the pancreas producing insufficient insulin to meet the needs of mother and baby in late pregnancy.

These causative factors don't, however, explain the recent big increase in gestational diabetes, which is likely to reflect increasing consumption of sugar and fast-absorbed carbohydrates, increased levels of environmental toxins and both insufficient sleep and insufficient exercise.

Gestational diabetes should not be ignored, as it can lead to birth problems and harm the health of the baby. It increases the risk of both stillbirth and pre-eclampsia (dangerously high blood pressure) and can lead to a large birth weight baby that needs to be delivered by Caesarean section. In addition, the baby is at greater risk of jaundice, breathing difficulties, low blood sugar and low blood calcium levels, polycythaemia (too many red cells in the blood) and heart function problems.

Gestational diabetes usually goes away immediately after the pregnancy, but around half of women who are diagnosed with gestational diabetes will develop type 2 (or sometimes type 1) diabetes within the next five years. That represents a massive seven-fold increase in risk, compared to women without gestational diabetes. The children of women with gestational diabetes are also at increased risk of developing obesity, impaired glucose tolerance and diabetes, as children or young adults (*Diabetes Care. 2007; 30(9):2287-2292*).

If you are pregnant or planning to become pregnant, you should take all possible steps to avoid gestational diabetes. First and foremost, cut down on sugar as much as you can and eat a low glycaemic load (GL) diet. This means a diet low in rapidly-absorbed carbohydrates, which will help you to control your blood sugar and won't push up your insulin levels. Make sure that you get plenty of sleep and take regular exercise. As far as possible, avoid cigarette smoke, household chemicals and other pollutants.

New research backs a low GL diet
for gestational diabetes

If you have already been given a diagnosis of gestational diabetes, don't panic. There is still plenty you can do to control the situation without drugs. It is now even more important to follow a low GL diet. The benefits of this approach have just been demonstrated in a clinical review of how diet affects pregnancy outcomes in gestational diabetes (*Curr Diab Rep. 2012 Oct 11. [Epub ahead of print]*). Scientific evidence consistently supports the advantages of, and has demonstrated no disadvantages of, a low GL diet for pregnant women with this condition.

You will need to work with your doctor, but don't be pressured or frightened into taking diabetes drugs or injecting insulin unless you are convinced that this is necessary, and if you do, work to reduce the dosage and come off medication as soon as possible.

The two drugs you are most likely to be offered are glibenclamide and metformin. Glibenclamide does not appear to cross the placenta and affect the baby, but it can cause hypoglycaemia and cholestasis (stopping the flow of bile) in the mother, along with digestive problems, nausea, faintness, tremor and weight gain. Metformin, on the other hand, causes less side effects in the mother but is able to cross the placenta and its safety for the baby has not been established.

Once the baby has arrived, gestational diabetes usually clears up. However, it means that you will have to take extra care to avoid diabetes in the future, both for yourself and for your growing child. As well as the measures mentioned above, breastfeeding for more than three months will also reduce your risk of subsequent diabetes, according to a new study from Germany (*Diabetes. 2012 Oct 15. [Epub ahead of print]*).

What this study also showed was that the risk of later diabetes in women who had experienced gestational diabetes was almost doubled in those women who had been given insulin treatment, compared with those who were treated through diet. This is another good reason not to be rushed into starting insulin or anti-diabetic drugs and to try diet and exercise first.

Technological breakthrough can help those battling with erratic blood sugar levels

Accumulation of pancreatic fat is common in diabetes, but getting a view of the organ has been difficult – until now...

US researchers at the University of Texas Southwestern Medical Center devised a way to use magnetic resonance spectroscopy (MRS) to examine the pancreas – a method that's non-invasive and doesn't expose the patient to harmful radiation.

In a recent trial, nearly 80 volunteers were examined using MRS. Results showed significantly higher amounts of pancreatic fat in subjects with symptoms of metabolic syndrome (a precursor of type 2 diabetes) compared to healthier subjects.

How doctors diagnose diabetes

Diabetes may be detected during a routine urine test when excess glucose is present.

When symptoms have drawn attention to the problem, blood tests such as a glucose tolerance test to look at insulin response (serial blood sugar levels are measured following a fixed dose sugary drink. A person with diabetes is unable to clear the blood sugar as quickly as a normal person), and an HbA1c test to look at long-term sugar levels, will confirm whether or not the underlying cause is diabetes.

Once diabetes is diagnosed, it's very important to attend regular check-ups, at least annually, in order to remain symptom-free and to prevent possible complications.

These check-ups include:

- Blood tests to monitor the level of glucose in the blood, including one called an HbA1c test which shows how well the diabetes has been controlled over the previous two to three months, cholesterol levels, and kidney function.

- Weight and blood pressure checks – blood pressure levels should be checked regularly to ensure they're at a safe level. Current guidelines recommend that someone with diabetes should have a blood pressure level below 130/80.

- Eye examinations – as diabetes can cause retinopathy (damage to the blood vessels in the retina at the back of the eyes). Laser treatment can be used to treat this when it's caught early enough.

- Examinations of the feet and nerves.

Helpful tips following a diabetes diagnosis

If you're diabetic and prescribed insulin, by law, you must inform the DVLA as soon as possible after you have been diagnosed. You should also inform the DVLA if you have diabetes as well as another relevant condition or complication, such as retinopathy (eye problems) or peripheral neuropathy (nerve damage to the legs or feet) – even if your diabetes is not treated with insulin. However, if your diabetes is treated by diet alone or diet and tablets, it is not necessary to inform the DVLA.

Wearing a medi-alert bracelet is also a good idea in case your blood sugar drops and you become confused or pass out or, alternatively, if your blood sugar skyrockets and you become confused. It also means that your condition can be identified straight away if you have an accident and fall unconscious.

If you receive a diabetes diagnosis you will normally be sent to visit a chiropodist, as good foot care is essential to prevent infections and ulcers developing, which may be slow to heal. You may also be allocated a diabetes specialist nurse. An appointment with a dietician may also be set up to advise you about a healthy diet and which foods are best for your condition... however, as you're about to discover in this report, this advice is often misguided and following it could do more harm than good!

Shocking rise in the number of diabetes-related complications

If not well controlled, diabetes-related complications – including heart disease, strokes, amputations, nerve damage, kidney failure and blindness – can develop. Worryingly, diabetes-related complications such as these are at a record high. The statistics make disturbing reading. For example, 80 per cent of people with diabetes will die from cardiovascular complications (*Diabetes in the UK, Diabetes UK, 2004 report*).

That's not all... 100 people a week in the UK have a limb amputated as a result of diabetes and 70 per cent of people die within five years of having an amputation as a result of diabetes (*Statistics taken from The Diabetic Foot Guide by the National Diabetes Support Team, 2006*). Plus, uncontrolled diabetes is the most common cause of blindness in people of working age.

An analysis carried out by Diabetes UK revealed that the rates of stroke and kidney failure in diabetes sufferers have surged in England. An audit of 1.9 million people with type 1 and type 2 diabetes found more than 13,000 had a stroke in 2009-10, a 57 per cent rise from 2006-7. And more than 7,000 had kidney failure, up 31 per cent from 2006-7.

Not only that but a recent survey by Diabetes UK suggested that almost a quarter of diabetes sufferers were unaware of having had their kidney function checked in the previous year, while 7 per cent had not had their blood pressure checked. Barbara Young, chief executive of the charity, said: "It is shocking that rates of strokes and kidney failure in people with diabetes are now at record levels and yet thousands of people are still not getting the health checks that can help prevent them.

"These figures are a reminder that all people with diabetes should have these checks every year, as this is the simplest and most effective way of reducing risk of complications such as stroke and kidney failure. We also need to get the message across to people with diabetes that they should demand these checks if they are not already getting them. Stroke and kidney failure are complications that hugely reduce quality of life for many people with diabetes, while the cost of treatment far exceeds that of the simple checks that can help prevent them developing in the first place".

Beware the potential dangers of blood pressure-lowering drugs for diabetics

If you have diabetes or metabolic syndrome, you will already know that it is important to keep your blood pressure well controlled. Having high blood pressure is one of several risk factors that can increase your chance of developing heart disease, a stroke or other complications. For many doctors, writing a prescription for a blood pressure-lowering drug seems the obvious solution – but the facts show that it can simply add to the risks.

Recently, the results of a clinical trial of the blood pressure drug aliskiren (Rasilez) were released. This drug was launched in 2007, with the usual puff of publicity, as the first of a new class of drugs, called direct renin inhibitors. Expectations were initially high, with the results of an animal study, published in 2008, showing that, as well as reducing blood pressure, aliskiren also reduced the artery-clogging lesions that can cause heart attacks and strokes (*J Clin Invest. 2008; 118(3):984-993*).

However, it didn't take long for doubts about aliskiren's safety to emerge. In November 2011, the manufacturer (Novartis) halted a large, international clinical trial of the drug, after finding that its use by people with diabetes led to an increase in strokes and kidney disease and to dangerously high levels of potassium in the blood. The full results of the study were published recently in the *British Medical Journal* (*BMJ. 2012; 344: e42*).

Far from being the breakthrough in blood pressure treatment that the manufacturers had claimed, the study showed that aliskiren was little better than placebo in reducing blood pressure. Just 17.9 per cent of patients taking the drug attained their target blood pressure level, compared with 16.8 per cent of those taking placebo. Even worse, while 2.7 per cent of the placebo group suffered a stroke during the two years that the trial had been running, the figure was 3.4 per cent for those taking aliskiren, an increase in risk of more than a third.

What can we learn from this? First, that the results of animal trials don't always apply to humans. And second, that it is often vulnerable patients who are the real guinea pigs.

Coeliac disease... or a drug side effect?

Aliskiren is far from being the only blood pressure drug to cause side effects. In another recent study, the medication olmesartan (Olmetec) was found to damage the gut in exactly the same way as coeliac disease, an autoimmune disorder that involves sensitivity to gluten (a protein found in wheat and some other grains) (*Mayo Clin Proc. 2012 Aug;87(8):732-8*). Doctors at the Mayo Clinic in the US found that some patients taking this drug developed chronic diarrhoea, bloating, abdominal pain and fatigue. Coeliac disease had been diagnosed in every case, but the patients failed to improve when they followed a gluten-free diet and blood tests showed they lacked the antibodies that are typical of the disease.

- Lose weight – most effectively by following a low glycaemic load (low GL) diet. Turn to page 57 for more details.

- Get regular exercise, to improve the efficiency of your heart and arteries.

- Limit alcohol consumption to 2 units a day, or less.

- Increase your intake of fibre and protein – easy to do with the low GL diet.

- Eat high-magnesium foods, such as almonds, pumpkin seeds, broccoli and dark chocolate.

- Increasing potassium may be even more important than reducing sodium – good sources are tomato paste, orange juice, spinach and dried fruit.

- Take a vitamin D supplement (2,000 IU a day).

- Eat plenty of oily fish, or take a fish oil supplement.

- Include garlic in your regular diet, or take garlic capsules.

- Try Alistrol, a Chinese herbal combination proven to reduce blood pressure.

• Are diabetics at greater risk of developing Alzheimer's?

Most people are aware of the increased risks of heart disease and stroke, and of problems with the eyes, kidneys and nervous system that come with a diabetes diagnosis. However, over the last few years another lesser-known association with diabetes has emerged, with a condition that some people fear more than any other – dementia.

A link between high blood sugar levels and reduced cognitive performance was suspected as early as 2004, in a study carried out at the University of California, in San Francisco (*Neurology. 2004; 63: 658–663*). The link was made when researchers analysed a mass of data collected over four years on more than 7,000 postmenopausal women, who had taken part in a trial of the drug raloxifene – an anti-oestrogen treatment for women with osteoporosis. They found more than double the incidence of cognitive impairment in women with diabetes or high fasting glucose levels, than in women with normal blood sugar readings.

The evidence linking type 2 diabetes and Alzheimer's disease risk is growing rapidly. The results of a 15-year Japanese study showed that the incidence of dementia, including Alzheimer's disease, was around 35 per cent higher in people over 60 with diabetes than in those with normal glucose tolerance (*Neurology. 2011 Sep 20; 77(12): 1126-34*). To put that in context, it isn't a huge increase in risk – from 20 per cent in non-diabetics to 27 per cent in diabetics – but it is part of a bigger picture of what happens in the brain when blood sugar and insulin levels are raised.

Recent research has been uncovering the mechanisms involved in the association between diabetes and dementia, although the situation seems far from simple. Magnetic resonance imaging studies have shown diabetic patients to have more constriction in brain blood vessels than control subjects and more atrophied brain tissue (namely a loss of neurons and the connections between them), particularly grey matter (*Diabetes Care. 2011 Nov; 34 (11): 2438-2441*). The grey matter includes regions of the brain involved in muscle control, sight, hearing, memory, emotions, and speech. Blood tests also showed high glucose levels to be strongly correlated with higher levels of inflammatory cytokines, which cause chronic inflammation, leading to blood vessel constriction, reduced blood flow and damage to brain tissue.

Because diabetes damages blood vessels and plays a role in hardening and narrowing the arteries in the brain, it puts sufferers at higher risk of vascular dementia. This is the kind that results from insufficient blood reaching the brain cells, which then become starved of oxygen and glucose, their fuel.

Your brain can become insulin resistant, too

As well as too much sugar, too much insulin also damages the brain in ways that can lead to Alzheimer's disease (*Curr Alzheimer Res. 2008 Oct; 5 (5): 438-447*). Oddly, though, too little insulin also seems to cause problems in the brain and insulin therapy has recently been put forward as a possible treatment for Alzheimer's disease. It appears that insulin resistance can occur in the brain, as well as in other types of body tissues, and that its effects there could interfere with signalling between brain cells, triggering a cascade of damaging events (*Biochem Soc Trans. 2011 Aug; 39 (4): 891-897*).

The good thing to come out of this research is a growing appreciation that keeping both blood sugar and insulin levels stable, which is of course the key to good diabetes control, may also prevent the development of Alzheimer's disease and other types of dementia. And there is no simpler or more effective means of doing this than through the food you eat.

In fact, scientists have already begun to investigate the effects of a low glycaemic load diet (for full details on this diet see page 57) in people with some degree of cognitive impairment. Glycaemic load (GL) is a measure of the overall effect that a meal or snack has on blood sugar levels. A study from Seattle, in the US, has found that, after just four weeks on a low GL and low saturated fat diet, visual memory improved, as did the markers for Alzheimer's disease, including beta-amyloid and tau protein in the cerebrospinal fluid (*Arch Neurol. 2011 Jun; 68 (6): 743-752*).

•   **Don't risk amputation due to diabetic Charcot foot**

Charcot foot syndrome, also known as Charcot neuroarthropathy, is a limb-threatening complication of diabetes, in which the bones of the foot and ankle soften and break. Charcot (pronounced shar-ko) foot is an enigmatic condition, whose accurate diagnosis and successful treatment continue to be a challenge to the medical profession. According to Dr Lee Rogers – lead author of an article in *Diabetes Care*, which summarised the report of an international task force of experts on the causes, diagnosis and treatment of Charcot foot syndrome – it's a problem that is not widely known or understood by most doctors.

It is vitally important for every person with diabetes to be aware of this and other foot problems associated with diabetes, so that they can recognise the risk and get any symptoms checked out thoroughly at an early stage.

Charcot foot has long been thought to be a result of diabetic neuropathy or nerve damage, but new research suggests that it may in fact be a separate inflammatory syndrome (*J Diabetes Complications. 2011; 25 (5): 320-324*). It causes calcium to be resorbed from the bones, in a localised form of osteoporosis. The bones are weakened enough to fracture and, with continued walking, the foot eventually changes shape. As the disorder progresses, the arch collapses, making walking very difficult and painful. Foot ulcers that refuse to heal are a distressing side effect of this condition.

In its early stages, when treatment is most likely to be successful, Charcot foot is notoriously difficult to diagnose, so there is every chance that your doctor will miss it, at least at first. One reason for this is that the little fractures in the foot bones often fail to show up on X-rays. In a 2005 study of patients referred to foot specialists, the condition was misdiagnosed in four out of every five patients, with most cases being mistaken for a sprain injury (*Diabet Med. 2005; 22 (12): 1707-1712*).

If caught early, Charcot foot can be helped by putting the foot in a cast and taking the weight off it. In the majority of cases, this seems to help the fractured bones to heal and prevents deformities. If you believe that you may have Charcot foot, don't rely on your GP's advice alone. Insist on seeing a specialist who has extensive experience of this condition, and do it as soon as you can.

Delayed diagnosis allows the condition to deteriorate to a point where immobilisation no longer helps and surgery may be considered instead. However, it seems that surgical outcomes may be hit-and-miss, according to a recent review (*Foot Ankle Int. 2012; 33(2):113-121*). A wide variety of surgical techniques has been tried out, but there has been no systematic review of their effectiveness. Drugs may not help much, either. Biphosphonates, which slow down bone resorption, have been used but, again, a recent review of their use found little supporting evidence that they aided recovery and some studies suggested that they may even delay healing (*Diabetologia. 2012; 55 (5): 1258-1264*).

What you can do to help prevent Charcot foot

As with most health problems, in the case of Charcot foot an ounce of prevention is worth a pound of cure. Keeping blood sugar levels under control is key, as with all aspects of diabetes, so it is important to keep to a low GL diet, make sure you always eat breakfast, get regular bouts of moderate exercise and don't forget to take any medication you may have been prescribed.

If you have diabetes, you need to take particular care of your feet. Some points to remember are:

- wash and examine your feet every day – look for swelling, tenderness, numbness and hot areas;

- wear comfortable and supportive shoes – never walk barefoot;

- be careful to avoid injury to your feet;

- keep your feet warm and dry;

- avoid long walks without taking a break.

If you are doing things right, it is unlikely that you will ever develop Charcot foot syndrome, but this really is a case of 'forewarned is forearmed'.

• **Why diabetics are at an increased risk of hearing loss and infertility**

Recent research has highlighted two diabetes-related health complications that are less well known about than others like cardiovascular disease, diabeteic foot ulcers and charcot foot – in fact, even your doctor may be unaware of them. These are hearing loss and male infertility.

A study carried out in Japan has found that people with diabetes have more than twice the incidence of hearing impairment than those without diabetes, after adjusting for other factors such as the effects of ageing or a noisy environment (*J Clin Endocrinol Metab. 2012 Nov 12 [Epub ahead of print]*). This latest study took the form of a meta-analysis of thirteen previous studies, involving more than 20,000 participants. The researchers believe that over time, high blood glucose levels can damage nerves and blood vessels in a part of the inner ear called the stria vascularis, diminishing the ability to hear.

In another recent study, scientists at Catania University in Italy have concluded that having diabetes could be a contributory factor in male infertility (*J Androl. 2012; 33 (2): 145-153*). They found that the oxidative stress associated with diabetes impairs sperm development and damages the nuclear and mitochondrial DNA in sperm cells. Diabetes may also cause reduced testosterone levels, leading to a low sperm count, while diabetic neuropathy seems to cause a loss of muscle tone in the seminal vesicles, bladder, and urethra, which may affect ejaculation. In addition, in people with type 1 diabetes, an autoimmune response may be responsible for impaired sperm production and the programmed death of sperm cells.

High insulin levels can lead to infertility in women, too

Women with type 1 diabetes are also at increased risk of infertility, according to recent research (*Hum Reprod Update. 2012; 18 (5): 568-585*). They may experience delayed puberty, be late in starting monthly periods, suffer menstrual problems (especially infrequent or irregular periods) and be prone to polycystic ovary syndrome (PCOS). In PCOS the ovaries produce a large number of immature follicles that fail to develop into fertile eggs and interfere with hormone balance, causing symptoms such as acne and excess body hair.

In fact, many experts believe that the main cause of PCOS, which is a common condition affecting between a quarter and a third of young women, is elevated insulin levels. High levels of insulin cause the ovaries to produce increased amounts of testosterone, leading to an imbalance of female sex hormones, such as luteinizing hormone and follicle stimulating hormone.

The messages from these research findings are clear. If you have diabetes, it is worth getting your hearing checked regularly in order to pick up any problems early (many high street opticians now offer this service). Conversely, if you experience an unexplained deterioration in your hearing and you haven't been diagnosed with diabetes, it would be worth talking to your doctor and getting your blood sugar level tested.

Similarly, if you have diabetes and are trying to start a family, it would be worthwhile getting the necessary checks on your fertility carried out, whether you are a man or a woman. If you are a woman who has been diagnosed as having PCOS, it is particularly important to follow a low-GL diet in order to keep your blood insulin level low. Following this dietary regime has been found to improve the regularity of menstrual cycles. Never skip breakfast and eat three low-GL meals a day, with healthy, low-GL snacks in between.

- **Keeping your blood sugar levels balanced is vital to ward off hypoglycaemia and hyperglycaemia**

One of the most common complications of diabetes is hypoglycaemia, which can lead to unconsciousness. Hypoglycaemia, or hypo, is the medical term for low blood glucose levels – that is a blood glucose level of less than 4 mmol/L. This is too low to provide enough energy for your body's activities. Hypos can happen when you are treated with insulin or some diabetes tablets. No matter how much you know about diabetes or how careful you are, if your diabetes is treated with certain medications, you are likely to experience some hypos. Similarly, there are certain tablets that will not cause hypos. Check with your doctor if you are unsure as to whether the treatment you are on is likely to cause hypos.

Very high blood glucose levels can cause hyperglycaemia. The World Health Organisation defines hyperglycaemia as:

- Blood glucose levels greater than 7.0 mmol/L (126 mg/dl) when fasting

- Blood glucose levels greater than 11.0 mmol/L (200 mg/dl) two hours after meals

Although blood sugar levels exceeding 7 mmol/L for extended periods of time can start to cause damage to internal organs, symptoms may not develop until blood glucose levels exceed 11 mmol/L.

The symptoms of hyperglycaemia are similar to the main symptoms of diabetes, but they are usually more severe and come on suddenly. They include extreme thirst, a dry mouth, blurred vision, drowsiness, and a need to pass urine frequently. Hyperglycaemia can occur for several reasons, including eating more carbohydrates than your body or medication can handle, being unwell, being mentally or emotionally stressed, and missing a dose of diabetic medication, tablets or insulin.

Left untreated, hyperglycaemia can cause a potentially life-threatening condition called diabetic ketoacidosis, where the body breaks down fat as an alternative source of energy. The body is unable to break down glucose due to the lack of insulin. This results in a build-up of acids in your blood, which will eventually cause unconsciousness and can lead to death if left untreated.

Self-monitoring is crucial

In addition to attending check-ups, it's also vitally important for diabetes sufferers to check their glucose levels regularly at home, so any problems can be detected and treated early. It's recognised that the sooner blood sugar levels are brought under control, the better the long-term prospects of preventing damage.

Self-monitoring glucose levels has the benefits of:

- Helping to detect when blood sugar levels may be too low (hypoglycaemia), or when medication is no longer effective and levels are starting to rise.

- Keeping blood sugar levels under control at times of illness, when these levels tend to rise, leading to hyperglycaemia.

- Giving an individual the confidence to be in control of their diabetes.

Most people are encouraged to measure their blood glucose at different times during the day or week. This is done by obtaining a small blood sample by pricking the skin. The sample is placed on to a test strip, which is then read by an electronic glucose test meter.

For people with type 2 diabetes who may find this type of testing difficult (in particular older people), a nurse can help perform this reading. Under certain circumstances, urine testing is simpler and provides satisfactory results.

Chapter 2

Mainstream medicine's approach to fighting diabetes

If you have been diagnosed with diabetes, the chances are you have been prescribed medication for it. Even if you have metabolic syndrome, which often precedes type 2 diabetes, you may be taking one of the following drugs:

Insulin. People with type 1 diabetes can't produce insulin, and have to inject themselves with one of the forms of insulin available as a pharmaceutical product. Some people with advanced type 2 diabetes also need to inject insulin.

Not all insulin is the same. There are four broad types, known as rapid-acting, short-acting, intermediate-acting and long-acting. Some people need it twice a day, some three times a day and some use an insulin pen to give themselves insulin just before meals.

It's important to work in partnership with your doctor in order to understand how these different forms of the drug work and what the best form (or combination of forms) is for you, since everybody reacts to them slightly differently.

How much insulin you need to inject, and how frequently, also depends on what you eat. Carbohydrates that are rapidly converted to glucose will push your blood sugar levels up faster and further than slow-release carbohydrates or proteins or fats. There's more on this subject in chapter 3, where you'll also discover how a nutritional approach could significantly reduce your need for injected insulin.

And you really do need to reduce it, since too much insulin pushes up your cholesterol level and blood pressure, damages your arteries and promotes weight gain. People who inject insulin also have a significantly higher risk of cancer, although the reason for this remains unclear

(*Diabetologia. 2011 Jul; 54(7): 1589-1592*).

Insulin delivery

Insulin injections can be administered using either a traditional needle and plastic syringe, or with an injection pen device, which many people find more convenient.

An automatic insulin pump is available, which means that fewer injections are needed. The needle is sited under the skin, and connected to a small electrical pump that attaches to a belt or waistband and is about the size of a pager. Inside is a reservoir of fast-acting insulin which is delivered continuously at an adjustable rate.

Oral insulin capsules herald a diabetes breakthrough

At present, the only way for people with type 1 or type 2 diabetes to take insulin is by injection. Insulin injections can be a harrowing experience and anybody who has to use them would love to be able to just swallow a capsule instead. Developing an oral form of insulin has been a 'holy grail' for the drugs companies for decades, but the obstacles seemed insurmountable. Now, though, it seems that the prize is almost within reach.

The problem with insulin is that, because it is a protein, it is easily broken down by enzymes in the digestive tract. Insulin is also a very large molecule, which means that it cannot be absorbed easily through the gut wall and circulated to the tissues where it is needed. These problems have stumped the drugs formulators for years, but the financial incentive is huge. Sales of an oral form of insulin have been predicted to be worth up to ten billion dollars a year worldwide.

Novo Nordisk are the world's biggest suppliers of injectable insulin and risk financial disaster if a competitor gets an oral form to the market before they do. Not surprisingly, they are putting massive resources into developing their own form of oral insulin and have already tested a prototype pill on animals and human volunteers.

The Israeli firm Oramed Pharmaceuticals also believes that it has developed a successful form of oral insulin that has shown good results in early trials. The formulation involves an enteric coated soft-gel capsule, which passes through the stomach unharmed and only disintegrates once it reaches the small intestine. An absorption enhancer then assists the insulin to cross the gut wall where it is transported to the liver like any other protein. Much of the insulin is broken down by the liver at this stage, but Oramed views this as a positive process that removes the risk of hypoglycaemia associated with injectable insulin.

Two biotechnology companies, Biocon and Tamarisk Technologies, have also developed oral delivery methods for insulin and are in licensing negotiations with pharmaceutical companies. Tamarisk Technologies has approached the problem in a unique way by designing what it calls 'serum-specific nano-encapsulate particles' that can trick the body cells into treating them as naturally-occurring molecules. Tamarisk say that their nano-sized particles are easily absorbed through the gut wall into the lacteal vessels, like fatty acids, and transported directly into the bloodstream, bypassing the liver.

Could oral insulin prevent type 1 diabetes?

As well as allowing people with diabetes to avoid having to inject insulin, the development of oral forms of insulin may help to protect people from getting type 1 diabetes in the first place. Type 1 diabetes is the autoimmune form of the disease, in which the patient's insulin-producing beta cells are destroyed by their own immune system. Scientists have discovered that people who have two specific kinds of antibodies, one of which is against insulin itself, are very likely to develop type 1 diabetes within five years. However, taking small daily doses of oral insulin could prevent this outcome.

A long-term study in Sweden recruited people with the two antibodies that predict type 1 diabetes and who also had a family member in whom the illness had been diagnosed (Diabetes Care. 2011; 34(7):1585). They were given daily doses of either oral insulin or placebo, which they continued to take for up to 10 years. At first, the results showed no difference between the two groups in terms of the numbers of participants who developed type 1 diabetes.

However, as the trial progressed, it became clear that oral insulin significantly delayed the onset of the disease. The researchers believe that the immune system becomes accustomed to the low daily doses of insulin in the gastrointestinal tract and that in time it is no longer perceived as a foreign substance. This line of reasoning is the same as for desensitisation for allergies, in which the dose of the substance that provokes the allergy is gradually increased.

Although these developments hold out much hope, particularly for those who suffer from, or are at risk of, type 1 diabetes, two things are certain. The first is that many years of testing and approval stages lie ahead before any new drug finally becomes available on prescription. The second is that, with a multi-billion dollar market at stake, you can guarantee (given their track record) that the drugs companies will be fighting dirty.

Inhaled insulin recently became available for treating people with a proven needle phobia or people who have severe trouble injecting. It was hoped that this would become a mainstay method of giving insulin, but initial results were not as impressive as hoped, and so this option is now usually reserved for those patients where all other treatment options have failed.

Artificial pancreas gives new hope
to type 1 diabetes sufferers

A research team at the University of Virginia in the US has now re-configured a standard smart phone to automatically monitor blood sugar levels and to deliver a shot of insulin as needed, so that it effectively acts as an artificial pancreas (*University of Virginia Health System (2012, March 19). Type 1 diabetes: Artificial pancreas approved for US outpatient testing*). The device has just received Food and Drug Administration (FDA) approval for outpatient clinical trials in America.

The artificial pancreas has been in development for several years, in collaboration with other universities in America and Europe, and initial outpatient trials in Italy and France have already shown promising results. When fully perfected and tested for reliability, this innovation could mark a major step forward for people with type 1 diabetes, relieving them from having to check their blood sugar levels regularly and inject insulin. Inability to control blood sugar effectively is the main cause of hospital admissions for people with type 1 diabetes. It also leaves them at increased risk of developing the potentially devastating complications of diabetes.

The University of Virginia work is not the only artificial pancreas project in the pipeline. Research has also been on-going in the UK, at Cambridge University and Addenbrooke's Hospital, on a similar kind of device, partly funded by Diabetes UK. Other institutions around the world are carrying out their own studies and developments. Medical companies are vying to be the first to market a cheap, reliable device that can operate for a long period without much attention.

Smart phone technology provides the
missing communication system

An artificial pancreas basically needs three things: a glucose monitor, an insulin pump and an 'algorithm' or computer programme to communicate between the two. The glucose monitor is a tiny sensor, inserted just under the skin, which checks blood glucose levels minute by minute. The insulin pump delivers measured doses of insulin to the body through a catheter, from a small insulin storage unit.

While glucose monitors and insulin pumps have both been around for some time and already help people with type 1 diabetes to get better control of their blood sugar, smart phone technology can now provide the vital link between them. It continuously picks up information on blood sugar levels from the glucose monitor and the algorithm works out whether it needs to tell the insulin pump to give more or less insulin. Basically, this is what a normally-functioning biological pancreas does.

Switching off the auto-immune attack

Other recent research has discovered why the body's immune cells, called T-cells, sometimes attack perfectly healthy cells causing autoimmune diseases like type 1 diabetes. Scientists have been studying a specific molecule, known as BIM, which is vital in regulating the normal death of T-cells (*Proc Natl Acad Sci U S A. 2012; 109(3):893-898*).

They found that when BIM was removed from T-cells, rather than being killed off and eliminated from the blood, the T-cells actually survived and were rendered inactive. These T-cells were no longer able to inflict the damage on insulin-producing cells in the pancreas that leads to type 1 diabetes. This discovery could be a first step in developing therapies for type 1 diabetes that can prevent auto-immune damage to the pancreas.

How type 2 diabetes drugs work

Metformin (brand name Glucophage) is the drug most commonly prescribed to type 2 diabetics, at least initially. Metformin works by increasing the insulin sensitivity of muscle cells, so that they take more glucose out of the bloodstream. It also reduces the amount of glucose produced by the liver. Even though metformin is generally considered to be 'safe', and may have anti-cancer effects, it has a major downside – it depletes the body of vitamin B12 (*Rev Assoc Med Bras. 2011 Jan-Feb; 57(1):46-49*). A low level of vitamin B12 means that homocysteine, a damaging protein associated with heart disease, nerve damage, cognitive decline and depression, can build up to dangerous levels. The longer you have been taking metformin, the more likely you are to be deficient in vitamin B12, so it makes sense to take a supplement of this and other B vitamins.

Sulphonylurea drugs encourage the pancreas to produce more insulin. The trouble is that most people with type 2 diabetes have too much insulin in their bloodstream anyway, it just isn't working properly! Along with side effects such as digestive problems, nausea, faintness, tremor and weight gain, you risk the cardiovascular problems that go along with high insulin levels. These drugs also become less effective the longer you take them.

Worse still, in a paper presented to the Endocrine Society's annual meeting in Houston, Texas, on 25 June 2012, researchers revealed three sulphonylurea drugs linked to an increased risk of death (*Science Daily 25 June 2012. http://www.sciencedaily.com/releases/2012/06/120625092236.htm*). After examining data on 24,000 patients with type 2 diabetes, they found that glipizide, glyburide and glimepiride increased mortality risk by more than 50 per cent when compared with metformin.

Alpha-glucosidase inhibitors are taken with a meal and slow down the absorption of carbohydrates in the gut, preventing a sharp rise in blood sugar (called postprandial hyperglycaemia). Their biggest drawback is their side effects, which include bloating, nausea, diarrhoea, and flatulence. Even if you can put up with these problems, these drugs are not very effective at reducing blood sugar levels.

The diabetes drug Pioglitazone has been found to increase the risk of bladder cancer

In June 2012, the *British Medical Journal* published a shocking study that showed the diabetes drug pioglitazone could almost double the risk of bladder cancer in people with type 2 diabetes (*BMJ. 2012; 344:e3645*). Bladder cancer is a dangerous disease. Just over 10,000 people are diagnosed with the condition every year and almost half of them die of it. Although this study's findings are damning, this is not the first time that pioglitazone has been linked to bladder cancer. Two reports published in 2011 in *Diabetes Care* had already set the alarm bells ringing.

One of these was an alert generated by the US Food and Drug Administration adverse event reporting system (*Diabetes Care. 2011; 34:1369-1371*), while the other was an interim analysis of a group of American users of the drug (*Diabetes Care. 2011; 34:916-922*). Both of these earlier studies suggested that pioglitazone may be associated with an increased risk of bladder cancer.

The latest study takes the 'maybe' out of it. Canadian researchers examined the UK general practice research database, which is the world's largest computerised collection of continuous primary care medical records, with complete information on more than 10 million patients. This massive number-crunching exercise produced unequivocal results. The use of pioglitazone is associated with a significantly increased risk of bladder cancer, up by 88 per cent in those taking it for two years or more. The standard line that 'more research is needed' won't wash this time.

That's not all… A study in 2005 had already linked pioglitazone with an increased risk of congestive heart failure (*Lancet. 2005; 366: 1279-1289*).

But don't expect to see pioglitazone banned any time soon, despite the evidence that it could be putting users' lives in danger. The European Medicines Agency still considers that 'the benefits outweigh the risks' and the pharmaceutical companies will fight tooth and nail to keep profitable thiazolidinedione drugs like this on the market, particularly while they are covered by time-limited patents.

New drugs, new dangers

Thiazolidinediones (also known as glitazones), act in a similar way to metformin, to improve insulin sensitivity. These drugs represent everything that is bad about the pharmaceutical industry. With the patent for metformin about to run out, meaning it would become less profitable, this group of drugs was aggressively developed and marketed, despite early indications that they caused weight gain, raised cholesterol levels and might carry increased risks of heart failure and osteoporosis.

Warning bells sounded in 2007, with a study showing the best-selling of these new drugs, called Avandia, was linked to an increase in heart attacks (*N Engl J Med. 2007 Jun; 356 (24): 2457-2471*). Instead of withdrawing the drug immediately, the manufacturer (Glaxo Smith Kline) carried out its own clinical trial, which claimed to show no such increase. But when that trial was scrutinised by the US Food and Drug Administration (FDA), they found it "seriously flawed". It was only in September 2010, after more studies, media campaigns and pressure from doctors themselves, that the European Medicines Agency recommended the suspension of Avandia.

The moral of this story has to be 'beware of new drugs', at least until they have been around for several years and any problems have had a chance to come to light. This is particularly relevant as another new class of diabetes drugs, called GLP-1 agonists, has recently become available. Already, studies have linked these drugs with increased risks of pancreatitis and pancreatic cancer (*Gastroenterology 2011; 141 (1): 150–156*).

Flawed intensive drug treatment study driven by commercial greed

The July 2012 issue of *Diabetes Care* featured a report on how a research team in America is advocating a one-size-fits-all approach for newly-diagnosed cases of type 2 diabetes, based on early and intensive treatment with insulin and anti-diabetes drugs (*Diabetes Care. 2012; 35(7): 1406-1412*).

The study, carried out at the University of Texas Southwestern Medical Centre, divided participants randomly into two groups. All of these patients had just been given a diagnosis of type 2 diabetes and none had previously received any treatment. Both groups were put on insulin and the anti-diabetes drug metformin, for the first three months. After that, one group took three types of diabetes medications daily, while the other continued the insulin and metformin treatment. This carried on for three and a half years.

The study found both these intensive treatment regimens to be equally effective. In both cases, diabetes patients maintained the function of their insulin-producing pancreatic beta-cells for the full duration of the study. Dr Ildiko Lingvay, one of the authors of the report, is quoted as saying: "The point is that whatever you choose, make sure it's intensive; we have shown that this preserves beta-cell function and that's the key in changing the course of the disease."

Can you see what's wrong here? It's almost like they are saying: "This group ate Smarties for a year while that group ate Maltesers and none of them broke a leg, so both types of sweet must be really good at preventing fractures!" There was no control group in this study. There was no comparison between the intensive drug treatment and, for instance, a regime that included diet, exercise and minimal use of drugs. Could that possibly have something to do with the fact that the study was part-funded by pharmaceutical company Novo Nordisk?

The researchers make the disclaimer that "Novo Nordisk played no role in the study design, conduct, analysis, preparation, or final approval". Yet Novo Nordisk is a major supplier of insulin medication and, as mentioned earlier, is currently competing with other drug companies to develop an insulin pill robust enough to survive the body's own defence mechanisms and deliver insulin to the bloodstream. That would free insulin users from the need to inject themselves and would instantly become a 'blockbuster drug', generating enormous profits for the company selling it. So, you can draw your own conclusions!

The researchers justify their proposed treatment regime by saying: "Unless dietary changes are significant and sustained long-term, diabetes is a progressive disease in which the body's ability to produce insulin declines". Yet, surely most diabetics given the choice would opt for changing to a healthier way of eating to control their diabetes rather than submitting to a lifetime of dependence on drugs that come with a litany of dangerous side effects?

It isn't even true that maintaining the insulin-producing capacity of the pancreas is the main issue with type 2 diabetes. For most people who have just been given a diagnosis of this condition, insulin resistance, leading to too much insulin in the bloodstream, is more likely to be a problem. Yes, the pancreas can eventually become 'exhausted' if insulin resistance and poor blood sugar control are allowed to continue, but putting every person who is diagnosed with type 2 diabetes straight onto a regime of insulin and drugs sounds like a strategy that is driven by commercial gain rather than by reason.

High levels of insulin in the bloodstream are not something any doctor should be aiming for, since they trigger a cascade of damaging effects in the body. The cells lining the arteries produce higher levels of clotting factors, which increase the risk of a heart attack. Fat accumulates, particularly in the abdominal region, which in turn makes the tissues even more insulin resistant. And if insulin levels stay high for long enough, they can actually kill the insulin-producing beta-cells in the pancreas. If that were not enough, high insulin levels have also been associated with prostate cancer in men, breast cancer in women, premature ageing, low sex hormone levels and loss of libido.

What every diabetic who requires a hospital stay needs to know

You might think that if you need to go into hospital, for any reason, you will at least be in the right place to get your diabetes properly looked after. Sadly, that could not be further from the truth, as a recently published major report shows. The National Diabetes Inpatient Audit 2011 took a snapshot of the care people with diabetes received in hospitals in England and Wales during one week in September 2011 (*National Diabetes Inpatient Audit 2011: Key findings about the quality of care of inpatients with diabetes in England and Wales. Health and Social Care Information Centre. May 2012*). Its findings make appalling reading.

During the seven days of the audit, almost one third of the patients experienced at least one medication error. These errors led to severe hypoglycaemia (low blood sugar) or diabetic ketoacidosis (a potentially life-threatening consequence of consistently high blood sugar) in a lot of cases.

According to Dr Gerry Rayman, the diabetes specialist leading the audit: "The majority of hospital doctors and ward nurses still do not have basic training in insulin management and glucose control". He was particularly critical of the cases in which people had developed diabetic ketoacidosis, saying: "Its occurrence is negligent and should never happen."

Patients' other main complaints were that they were not allowed as much control over their own diabetes as they would have liked, and that the hospital did not provide the right type of food to help them manage their diabetes.

So, what can you do to make sure you do not become a victim of the overstretched, under-trained, inadequate and occasionally downright incompetent NHS care provision for people with diabetes? The following 10 tips can help:

- Be aware of the signs and symptoms of diabetes; if you think you may have diabetes, talk to your doctor.

- If you have been diagnosed with diabetes, ask your doctor to explain the disease and the treatment options to you in depth; if you are not satisfied, ask for a referral to a specialist.

- Every person with diabetes should get a planned programme of nine recommended checks each year; make sure you get these tests regularly.

- Follow a low glycaemic load diet and cut right back on sugar and simple carbohydrates.

- Get regular exercise and lose weight if you need to.

- If you have to go into hospital, take with you any medications you have been given and any treatment plan or test results from your doctor or specialist, to show to hospital staff.

- Check everything, especially medications you are asked to take – mistakes are commonplace on hospital wards – and don't be afraid to question anything that doesn't seem right.

- Ask hospital staff to explain to you what medication you are being given and why; if you are not happy, insist on talking to a consultant or senior doctor.

- Ask family and friends to bring in low GL food items for you, if the hospital menu is unsuitable.

> - If you feel that your blood sugar levels are not being properly controlled, say so and ask to see a senior member of the medical staff if necessary.

If you are taking any diabetes drugs or other medications, you should always be aware of potential side effects and let your doctor know of any unusual symptoms. In particular, if you are taking pioglitazone or a related drug, discuss the options for changing to a safer alternative and immediately report any blood in your urine or any bladder symptoms, such as pain when passing urine or feelings of urgency.

Sadly, mainstream diabetes treatment all-too-often appears to be dominated by a lucrative 'sickness industry', fuelled by the profits from risky drugs, while vulnerable patients are the guinea pigs in a grotesque experiment. Medication should be viewed as a last resort for people with diabetes rather than the mainstay of treatment as it currently is. As you're about to discover in the coming chapters, the right diet, regular exercise and some specific nutritional and herbal supplements can do a great deal to reduce the need for drugs.

Chapter 3

Following a healthy diet and taking more exercise can be more effective than metformin

It's hardly ground-breaking news that being overweight (80 per cent of diabetics are overweight) and having a sedentary lifestyle are two of the main risk factors that contribute to type 2 diabetes, in addition to smoking. Yet, the fact that simple dietary and lifestyle changes can make a massive difference to your likelihood of developing the disease – and can even fully reverse type 2 diabetes in its early stages – is all-too-often overlooked by the medical mainstream, who seem to favour the quick fix of prescription drugs.

Given the choice between following a healthy eating and exercise programme or a lifelong reliance on drugs, with all their attendant side-effects, most people would probably opt for the former... especially given that a large placebo-controlled study of 3,234 overweight participants (average age of 51) with impaired glucose (who were classed as being at risk of developing diabetes), found that lifestyle changes (dietary modifications plus regular exercise) were almost twice as effective as the drug Metformin, in reversing symptoms (*US National Institute of Health – The Diabetes Prevention Programme; New England Journal of Medicine, 7 February 2002*).

During the study, which formed part of the Diabetes Prevention Programme, those following a healthy diet and taking 150 minutes of exercise a week were found to reduce their risk of type 2 diabetes by 58 per cent, compared to those taking the drug metformin who only reduced their risk of the disease by 31 per cent in comparison.

Patients in the lifestyle modification group achieved an average weight-loss of 7 per cent, which was sustained throughout the study. Not only were lifestyle changes shown to prevent or delay the development of type 2 diabetes, but they also restored normal glucose levels in many of the patients (50 per cent of those with impaired glucose tolerance go on to develop type 2 diabetes). The researchers concluded that type 2 diabetes can be prevented by following a healthy diet and doing more exercise.

Reap the benefits of a low glycaemic load way of eating

For years doctors and dieticians advised diabetics to base every meal on starchy carbohydrates, go easy on the protein and keep fats to a minimum. While this way of thinking is gradually beginning to change, as evidence mounts up to show how this way of eating actually contributes to high blood sugar levels, the concept of a 'food pyramid', with carbohydrates as its broad base, has become ingrained in medical doctrine and is still defended by many in the medical profession even today.

Interest in diets that limit fluctuations in blood sugar has been gaining ground. In 2009, a meta-analysis of eleven separate, randomised, placebo-controlled clinical trials was published under the prestigious Cochrane Database of Systematic Reviews, which maintains the most rigorous scientific standards. The review concluded that: "A low-GI diet can improve glycaemic control in diabetes without compromising hypoglycaemic events" (*Cochrane Database Syst Rev. 2009 Jan 21;(1):CD006296*).

This means that a low carbohydrate diet will help you to control your blood sugar and won't cause you to become hypoglycaemic. GI stands for 'glycaemic index', a measure of the speed at which a carbohydrate raises blood sugar levels. More useful in practice is the idea of 'glycaemic load' (GL), which also takes account of how much of a carbohydrate is in a food and what portion size is being eaten.

Was Dr Atkins right all along?

The late Dr Atkins, who caused a great deal of controversy by advocating a low carbohydrate diet, was well ahead of his time when he wrote a chapter in his *New Diet Revolution* book entitled: 'Insulin – the hormone that makes you fat'. Long before the term 'metabolic syndrome' had been coined, Dr Atkins was describing how a high carbohydrate diet leads to insulin resistance and a pre-diabetic 'diet-related disorder', involving high insulin levels, poor blood sugar control, high blood pressure, escalating cholesterol levels, fatigue and weight gain.

What is more, Dr Atkins recognised, over 20 years ago, that diets high in carbohydrates were to blame for what he realised was a growing epidemic of diabetes. And he saw that when people diagnosed with type 2 diabetes were put on the standard high carbohydrate, low fat diets, their diabetes worsened to the point that their doctors then prescribed insulin or other drugs. In 1992, Dr Atkins wrote: "I hate to be so cynical as to suggest that proper diet might adversely affect the thoroughly profitable administration of insulin and oral diabetic drugs, but I will certainly say that if sugar were denounced from the scientific pulpits as if it were sin, it would seriously compromise a mutually supportive food and pharmaceutical industrial culture."

Whether you have type 1 or type 2 diabetes, or suspect you have metabolic syndrome or insulin resistance, your primary aim has to be to keep your blood sugar level as stable as possible and to keep your need for insulin (injected or produced by your pancreas) low. The best tool at your disposal is your diet – and a low GL diet is definitely the way to go. A massive European study involving almost 38,000 people from 21 to 70 years of age recently showed a clear correlation between a high GL diet and diabetes risk (*Am J Clin Nutr. 2010 Oct; 92(4):905-11*). A diet high in starch was also linked to increased diabetes risk, sinking once and for all the outdated idea that eating starchy carbohydrates will help you control your blood sugar.

Unfortunately, despite the overwhelming evidence in favour of reducing glycaemic load, the charity Diabetes UK has been slow to change its advice. Its website still says: "Base your meals on starchy carbohydrate foods such as bread, pasta, potatoes, noodles, rice, chapatis and breakfast cereals. These fill you up, give you energy and help you to control your blood glucose levels." To be fair, Diabetes UK has shown some recognition of the value of a low

GL eating plan for diabetes and now says that a diet where less than 45 per cent of calories come from carbohydrates may be suitable in the short term, for people with type 2 diabetes who need to lose weight. However, Diabetes UK stresses it is not advocating this diet for everyone and they consider there is little evidence to support its use for people with type 1 diabetes, which is an autoimmune condition. This seems extremely short-sighted, to say the least.

The fact is that a low GL way of eating can benefit anyone with metabolic syndrome and those with type 1 or type 2 diabetes. It is central to putting you in control of your blood sugar and keeping your insulin levels stable... it can even reduce your reliance on medication and reduce your risk of diabetes-related complications. It can also help you lose any excess weight – another diabetes risk factor. If that weren't reason enough to switch to a low GL eating plan then there's always increased energy levels and healthier cholesterol and blood pressure readings to look forward to.

Glycaemic load is an accurate indication of how something you eat will affect your blood sugar level. Learning which foods have a low glycaemic load (GL) and eating them in preference to high-GL foods is a basic lifestyle tool for anybody who has type 1 or 2 diabetes or metabolic syndrome. Refined carbohydrates, like white bread and pasta, should be avoided as much as possible as they have a high glycaemic load and are rapidly converted to sugar in your digestive tract. When you absorb large amounts of sugar (as glucose), your pancreas is forced to produce large amounts of insulin in order to deal with it. Some of this glucose can be used to produce energy, but high amounts cause weight gain and low energy levels.

If excessive amounts of carbohydrates continue to be eaten, your blood sugar levels will continue to rise and can cause your cells to become insulin resistant... this puts you at high risk of developing type 2 diabetes. For the same reason, you should steer clear of sugar too.

A low GL diet does not need to be particularly low in carbohydrates – it's the type of carbohydrate that is important. So, you can still eat bread, but make it whole wheat with rye, and don't overdo it. Or try oatcakes instead. Have porridge oats for breakfast instead of corn flakes and if you want to eat pasta, make sure it's the whole wheat kind. Replace potatoes with squash, swede, carrots or beetroot. Try quinoa or buckwheat instead of rice.

Opt for high fibre foods and protein, which produce a much lower insulin response than refined carbs. Other foods to consume more of are vegetables, beans and pulses, which release sugar into your bloodstream at a slower rate (*Balance Diabetes UK Nov/Dec 2001*).

Eating regularly during the day (little and often is the rule of thumb here) and having a low-GL breakfast every morning is also important – several studies have shown that people who don't eat a proper breakfast tend to have poorer appetite control and blood sugar control throughout the day. People who are not already diabetic and who regularly skip breakfast are at an increased risk of developing type 2 diabetes, according to a new study from Harvard Medical School.

This is the basic dietary strategy for keeping your blood sugar levels stable, preventing or managing insulin resistance and reducing your reliance on insulin and diabetes drugs.

Regular exercise helps stabilise your blood sugar levels

Regular exercise, not smoking, drinking alcohol in moderation and keeping to an ideal weight are also important for keeping your blood sugar levels stable and can help prevent the complications of diabetes, such as heart disease. Smoking should be completely avoided since it greatly increases the risk of many health problems, including damage to the blood vessels (already a concern for diabetics)... even passive smoking has been linked with the development of type 2 diabetes (*Endocrine Society 94th Annual Meeting. Houston, Texas. 23-26 June 2012*).

When it comes to alcohol, heavy drinking can reduce the body's sensitivity to insulin, which can trigger type 2 diabetes, and can lead to high blood pressure and weight gain. Plus, diabetes sufferers should never drink on an empty stomach because this can cause hypoglycaemia.

Exercise is vital as it increases the insulin sensitivity of your cells so less insulin is required to transport glucose into them. The good news is that it's not necessary to spend hours down the gym; just 30 minutes of brisk walking or cycling three or four times a week is adequate. Obviously, you should talk to your doctor before making any drastic change to your diet or starting an exercise regimen, particularly if you are overweight or obese.

The importance of losing any excess weight can't be emphasised enough for getting your blood sugar levels under control...

• How obesity causes type 2 diabetes

In addition to impaired glucose metabolism, type 2 diabetes is also characterized by impaired fat metabolism. When blood sugar levels are high, the body does whatever it can to protect the brain and other vital organs from the toxic effects of too much glucose, initially loading it into muscle cells, then converting it to fat for storage in fat cells (or adipose tissue as scientists call it).

We used to think of body fat as being like lard – an inert, white substance that we just lug around with us. We now know that fat is far from inert. In fact, adipose tissue plays a crucial role as an endocrine organ and secretes numerous bioactive substances, collectively known as adipokines, which have profound effects on our physiology. Obesity is now recognized as a chronic inflammatory disease in its own right, which profoundly affects carbohydrate and fat metabolism, immune function and cardiovascular disease risk (*Int J Inflam 2011; 2011:529061. Epub 2011 Aug 3*).

Visceral fat, the kind that collects around your body organs, produces more adipokines than subcutaneous fat, the kind that lies just under your skin. The amount of visceral fat you have is a pretty reliable indicator of insulin sensitivity, impaired glucose tolerance, high blood pressure and high cholesterol and triglyceride levels.

The link between body fat and insulin resistance is becoming clearer

So, just how does being fat cause type 2 diabetes? The irony is that some of the adipokines produced by fat cells, such as the hormones leptin and adiponectin, are known to improve insulin sensitivity, suppress appetite, increase metabolic rate and increase physical activity (*Mol Med 2008; 14 (11-12): 741-51*). Your body is in fact trying to regulate itself and make you slimmer.

But, as the amount of adipose tissue increases, consistently high levels of adipokines in the bloodstream cause this control system to become overloaded. The receptors no longer respond, so your muscle cells become less sensitive (i.e. more resistant) to insulin and you don't know when to stop eating, you can't burn fat and you can't find the energy to exercise. It's a vicious circle. The result is insulin resistance, metabolic syndrome and, eventually, type 2 diabetes.

This is why controlling your weight is important in avoiding or managing type 2 diabetes. And it shows you why it is important to take action at an early stage, before your fat cells take over control of your metabolism. Of course, losing those extra fat stores is a good thing however heavy you are, but it is a whole lot easier to do if you don't let it get out of hand.

There's one kind of fat that actually helps you to lose weight!

The kind of fat that produces adipokines is called 'white adipose tissue', but there is another sort, called 'brown adipose tissue' that until fairly recently was thought to be found only in infants. New imaging technology has revealed, though, that this special kind of fat cell is also present in most adults. What gives it its brown colour is its high concentration of mitochondria, the energy-producing centres inside the cells. Brown adipose tissue doesn't just store fat, it actively burns it. The more brown fat people have, the less likely they are to be obese.

Now scientists at the University of California have discovered a protein that is able to convert white fat cells to brown fat cells (*Cell Metabolism 2012; 15(3):395*). What is more, they have found that a class of drugs called PPAR-gamma ligands stabilise this protein, leading to its accumulation inside cells. This essentially 'throws a genetic switch' and converts the white fat cells to brown – at least in mice.

The question remains whether it is possible to do this in people as well, and if so, how. The development of a safe and effective medication that can make this amazing conversion is probably still several years away. In the meantime, we shall have to rely on our old friends' diet (a low GL one) and exercise to help keep our weight down and keep type 2 diabetes at bay. In addition, CLA (conjugated linoleic acid) can also help shift those extra pounds. Taking 2,500mg of CLA each day helps your body to burn fat more effectively and builds muscle tissue (which in turn burns more fat). Another benefit of CLA is that it helps maintain healthy blood glucose and cholesterol levels.

Losing weight by following a low GL diet not only has important implications in the fight against diabetes but may help ward off dementia too...

- **Study shows type 2 diabetes starts in the brain and can be triggered by overeating**

Anybody with diabetes or metabolic syndrome knows that what they eat will affect their blood sugar and that if they eat too much of the wrong things they will put on weight. That much is common sense, but now scientists in New York have found how overeating could cause a malfunction in insulin signalling in the brain, leading to obesity and diabetes (*J Biol Chem. 2012; 287 (39): 33061-33069*).

What the researchers discovered, in a series of experiments on laboratory rats, was that a high calorie, high fat diet first damages the brain, starting a downward spiral that eventually leads to insulin resistance in the rest of the body, weight gain and type 2 diabetes.

It had already been established, from earlier experiments, that a function of insulin in the brain is to suppress the signals that the brain sends to the body's fat cells to stimulate the release of fatty acids into the bloodstream. The new study found that increasing the rats' intake of calories by 37 per cent, by adding lard to their diet, caused their brain cells to become insulin resistant in just three days. This led to increased brain signalling to the fat cells, resulting in elevated blood levels of both fatty acids and insulin, compared to rats fed a normal diet.

High levels of fatty acids in the bloodstream have been found to induce inflammation, which in turn leads to insulin resistance in the muscle cells, the main metabolic problem in type 2 diabetes. Fatty acids also increase glucose production in the liver which raises blood sugar levels. So, if the results of this study apply to humans, simply eating too much could lead to increased levels of fats, sugar and insulin in the bloodstream, the perfect recipe for type 2 diabetes.

Related research, presented to the annual meeting of the Society for Neuroscience in October 2012, has found that a high-sugar diet also affects the insulin receptors in rats' brains in the same way and may dull spatial learning and memory skills (*Neuroscience 2012, New Orleans, 13-17 October 2012. http://www.sfn.org/AM2012*). However, omega-3 fatty acids, such as those found in fish oils, were able to reduce this effect and maintain insulin sensitivity in the brain. Omega-3 fatty acids were already known to reduce insulin resistance in muscle cells, but this is the first time that the effect has also been demonstrated in the brain.

High carb, low fat diets raise the
risk of cognitive impairment

The results of these animal studies tie in with the newly-released findings of a long-term evaluation of diet and cognitive impairment in humans. Researchers at the prestigious Mayo Clinic in the US monitored the diets and cognitive performance of 1,230 people aged 70 to 89, over a period of four years. They found that those with the highest carbohydrate and sugar intakes were most likely to develop mild cognitive impairment (*J Alzheimers Dis. 2012; 32 (2): 329-339*).

A bigger surprise is that those participants whose diets were highest in fat or protein, on the other hand, actually reduced their risks of cognitive impairment, by 42 per cent and 21 per cent respectively. When total fat and protein intake were taken into account, people with the highest carbohydrate intake were almost four times more likely to develop mild cognitive impairment than those eating the least carbohydrates. Taken together, these results really blow a hole in the 'low fat, high complex carbohydrates' dietary advice that is still being propagated for people with diabetes.

Cognitive impairment and dementia, including Alzheimer's disease, are now firmly linked with insulin resistance in the brain. Another new study has confirmed that insulin resistance leads to brain atrophy, less 'grey matter' and poorer cognitive performance in late middle-aged adults (*Diabetes Care. 2012 Oct 15. [Epub ahead of print]*). If you ever doubted just how closely diabetes and dementia are linked or were reluctant to ignore the official line on a high-carb diet for diabetes, hopefully these new research results will convince you otherwise.

It really can't be emphasized enough that reducing the glycaemic load (GL) of your diet – that is, the impact it has on your blood sugar levels – is the surest way to avoid both type 2 diabetes and Alzheimer's disease, and even to completely reverse type 2 diabetes for the majority of people with the condition. Avoiding added sugar, foods made with white flour, potatoes, white rice and other starchy items is a fairly obvious way of keeping the GL of a meal low.

Gut bacteria linked to obesity and type 2 diabetes

You may not think too often about the 'bugs' that live in your gut, but you are providing a home to around one hundred trillion microbes, mainly in your colon. The 'gut flora', as they are called, include bacteria, fungi and various other single-celled organisms. This complex community of microbes normally exists in a mutually beneficial relationship with your body.

The gut flora perform many useful functions, such as producing vitamin K and biotin, regulating the immune system and suppressing the growth of harmful bacteria.

A new study from the University of Maryland School of Medicine in the US, though, has shown that some bacteria in the human gut have a more sinister role; they are linked to the development of obesity, metabolic syndrome and type 2 diabetes (*PLoS One. 2012; 7(8): e43052. Epub 2012 Aug 15*).

The study analysed the gut bacteria in 310 members of the Old Order Amish in Pennsylvania. Interestingly, the results showed that each person had one of three different communities of gut flora, each characterised by a dominant type of bacteria. However, it was not the type of gut flora community that was linked to obesity and metabolic syndrome, but instead differing levels of 26 less abundant bacterial species.

So, how can gut bacteria make you fat and cause metabolic syndrome and diabetes? The research team also found an apparent link between the gut bacteria they identified and inflammation, which is believed to be a factor in obesity and many other chronic diseases. Other recent research has helped to reveal what may be going on (*Mol Syst Biol. 2010 Jul; 6: 392*).

'Leaky gut', inflammation and adipokines promote metabolic syndrome

Bacterial cell walls contain compounds called lipopolysaccharides. Some bacteria (the ones that make you fat) have a lot more of these compounds in their cell walls than others. When the bacteria die and their cell walls break down, the lipopolysaccharides are released. These then trigger receptors in the gut lining, causing the normally tight junctions between the epithelial cells to open up, so allowing the lipopolysaccharides to slip through and get into the bloodstream. This condition is often referred to as 'leaky gut syndrome'.

Once in the blood and tissue fluid, lipopolysaccharides provoke a strong reaction from the immune system, resulting in inflammation. In people who have a lot of the offending bacteria in their gut, this situation becomes chronic and the on-going, low-grade inflammation promotes both the formation of adipose (fatty) tissue and the deposition of fat within it.

This adipose tissue doesn't just sit there. It becomes an active endocrine organ, producing hormones called adipokines, which as mentioned earlier, promote further inflammation and influence sugar and fat metabolism, leading to insulin resistance, high blood levels of sugar and insulin, the deposition of cholesterol in the arteries and high blood pressure – in other words, metabolic syndrome.

What can you do to avoid this situation? Cutting down on sugar and saturated fat is one way, since both have been shown to favour harmful gut bacteria and increase the transport of lipopolysaccharides across the gut wall. Looking after your 'good' bacteria is important, since they will suppress the growth of the kinds that are guilty of provoking inflammation. Here are 10 things you can do to promote a healthy balance of gut flora:

- Don't eat red meat more than once or twice a week;

- Have fibre-rich vegetables or salads with all main meals and snack on fresh berries and nuts between meals;

- Eat foods containing 'prebiotic' soluble fibre, which feeds beneficial gut flora, such as chicory, leeks, onions, Jerusalem artichokes and garlic;

- Eat fish (preferably oily fish) two or three times a week;

- Have 'live', unsweetened yoghurt daily or take a probiotic supplement;

- Avoid processed foods and refined carbohydrates;

- Stress hormones are bad for your gut bacteria, so avoid chronic stress as far as possible and find ways to de-stress your life;

- Avoid taking antibiotics and other medications unless they are essential;

- Since food allergies, particularly to wheat, can cause 'leaky gut syndrome', if you suspect you have one, get it checked out;

- Get appropriate (preferably natural) treatment for any chronic infection, including gut parasites, that may be disrupting your gut flora.

- **Just because you're thin, don't think you can't get diabetes**

Practically every report about diabetes nowadays advises sufferers and those who want to reduce their risk of developing the condition to lose weight. The twin epidemics of diabetes and obesity are inextricably linked as far as the media are concerned. You could be forgiven for thinking that, if you are not overweight, you've got nothing to worry about. But you'd be wrong.

It is quite true that around 80 per cent of diabetes sufferers are overweight; that is to say, they have a body mass index (BMI) of more than 25. But not all fat people develop diabetes and not all diabetics are fat. So, what about the minority we never hear about – the ones who stay thin but still get diabetes?

About 20 per cent of the three million people currently diagnosed with diabetes in the UK are of normal weight or underweight. But it is estimated that one third of all diabetics remain undiagnosed and a significant proportion of these 'hidden' sufferers are likely to be thin, because they are under the impression that 'only fat people get diabetes'.

To work out what is going on, it is important to understand that type 2 diabetes is not a disease, it's a symptom. Any factor, or combination of factors, that interferes with the body's normal control of blood sugar levels can lead to type 2 diabetes. It is just as important for thin people to keep their blood sugar under control as it is for those who are overweight.

You may have difficulty with blood sugar control for genetic reasons; it has been found that the children of people with type 2 diabetes are much more likely to develop insulin resistance (*N Engl J Med. 2004; 350 (7): 664-671*). Non-alcoholic fatty liver disease, a condition that is becoming ever more prevalent in industrialised societies, can also lead to metabolic syndrome and type 2 diabetes (*Arterioscler Thromb Vasc Biol. 2008; 28 (1): 27-38*). Chronic inflammation and stress are further contributing factors.

Is reactive hypoglycaemia putting you at risk of type 2 diabetes?

Even if you consider yourself to be reasonably fit and of normal weight, things can still go wrong with your blood sugar control. The commonest cause is called 'reactive hypoglycaemia'. This happens when you eat something that pushes your blood sugar up very fast, such as a jam doughnut or a big bowl of sugary breakfast cereal.

Your body knows that high blood sugar is very damaging and has rapid response control mechanisms to counteract it. So, your pancreas releases a surge of insulin, to bring it back down, but it over-compensates so that your blood sugar becomes too low, or hypoglycaemic. The reason your blood sugar control mechanism doesn't work perfectly in this situation is that it evolved when we were hunter-gatherers and jam doughnuts just weren't on the menu!

Low blood sugar makes you feel sleepy, irritable, anxious, forgetful and unable to concentrate. Some people even experience mood swings, abnormal thoughts and 'drunken' behaviour. That is because your brain has an absolute need for glucose. When it isn't getting enough, another control mechanism kicks in and your liver converts its stores of glycogen into glucose to raise blood sugar.

Reactive hypoglycaemia is often the first step on the slippery path to type 2 diabetes, a journey that can take up to 10 years. But it won't show up when your doctor orders a fasting blood glucose test, the standard screening procedure for diabetes, because after several hours without eating your levels will have returned to normal. By the time your blood sugar control has deteriorated to the point that you get an abnormal reading with this test, diabetes is already a reality.

Fortunately, the solution to the problem is simply to plan your eating and lifestyle to prevent those wild swings in blood sugar levels. A low GI diet provides the basis of this. In addition:

- Never skip breakfast

- Have protein, fibre and low GI carbs at every meal

- Avoid sugary and starchy snacks and multiple teas and coffees

- Eat little and often – five small meals a day often works best

- Don't have your main meal late in the evening

- Remember to drink plenty of water

- Take regular, moderate exercise

• **How dietary changes can benefit type 1 diabetes sufferers**

Around 90 per cent of diabetes sufferers have type 2 diabetes, a metabolic problem that usually involves insulin resistance. There is plenty of information around for type 2 diabetics to help them manage their condition with diet and lifestyle. However, if you are part of the 10 per cent minority with type 1 diabetes – an autoimmune condition in which the body's immune system destroys the insulin-producing cells of the pancreas – you may feel that there is nothing that you can do apart from continue to inject insulin regularly and monitor your blood sugar levels. Well, that's a common misconception.

The first question we should ask about type 1 diabetes is: Why does the immune system malfunction and attack the body? Your doctor may tell you that it's all down to the genetic lottery and you were unlucky enough to inherit a faulty gene. But that is only part of the problem. The rapidly increasing incidence of type 1 diabetes in western societies cannot be attributed to genetics alone. Something else must be driving it.

Scientists have recently found that type 1 diabetes is part of an interrelated complex of autoimmune conditions that also includes coeliac disease, rheumatoid arthritis, and multiple sclerosis (*Genome Med. 2012 Jan 27; 4 (1): 6*). There is increasing evidence that, in all of these conditions, a genetic susceptibility only becomes a reality if the relevant gene is 'switched on' by an environmental trigger. In many cases, the trigger is food.

With coeliac disease, the trigger food is a protein in wheat gluten, called gliadin. New research at the Royal Hallamshire Hospital in Sheffield has discovered that people with type 1 diabetes, who also have coeliac disease, have poorer blood sugar control and a higher incidence of complications than other type 1 diabetics. Following a gluten-free diet led to better blood sugar and blood fat profiles and less incidence of diabetes-related kidney damage in these patients (*Diabetes Care. 2011 Oct; 34 (10): 2158-63*).

Because the immune system is still developing during the first few years of life, most nutritional practitioners advise against introducing wheat or cow's milk products into a baby's diet before the age of 12 months. These foods frequently induce immune reactions. Animal studies suggest that wheat-based diets can promote the development of type 1 diabetes and there is some evidence that the same may be true of cow's milk (*Cytokine. 2003 Feb 7; 21 (3): 149-54*).

For people who are already living with type 1 diabetes, these findings are relevant because damage to the insulin-producing cells in the pancreas (called beta cells) is not an all-or-nothing occurrence. Many type 1 diabetics still have some beta cell function and may be able to prevent further damage by following the right diet. Once the immune system is no longer attacking these cells, there is also the possibility that they could regenerate and start to produce some insulin again.

The practical message for people with type 1 diabetes is twofold. First, strengthen your immune system. Second, cut out foods that may trigger an immune reaction.

Foods that support a strong, properly functioning immune system are mainly fresh plant and animal foods in their natural state. Particularly good are oily fish, leafy green vegetables, berries, seeds, garlic, mushrooms, oats and green tea. As a general rule, the more processed a food is, the worse it is for your immune system. Taking regular, moderate exercise in the fresh air, dealing with stress and getting enough sleep are also important.

Although wheat and dairy foods may be the prime suspects, many other foods can cause allergies or intolerances. If you suspect that you have problems of this kind, it may be worth getting tests done. Some allergy testing is available on the NHS and you should talk to your doctor in the first instance. If you want a full spectrum of food intolerance testing, you will need to arrange this privately, in which case make sure that you get proper blood tests (called IgG tests) done by a reputable UK laboratory.

Type 1 diabetics can also benefit from following a low glycaemic load (low GL) diet. Eating a poor diet can result in insulin resistance developing in people who inject insulin, as much as in those who produce their own. A low GL diet on the other hand could mean that you can cut back your injected insulin by as much as 50 per cent and benefit from reduced risks of cancer and heart disease as a bonus.

The key for people with type 1 diabetes is to make changes to the diet very gradually and monitor blood sugar carefully while doing so. Work together with your doctor to agree reduced doses of insulin as your blood sugar levels start to drop. Make changes to breakfast and lunch first, so that you are aware of their effects while you are awake. Cutting back on caffeine and alcohol will also help.

• Epigenetics holds new hope for diabetes sufferers

An incredible revolution in scientific thinking could bring big benefits for people with diabetes or metabolic syndrome, but since it doesn't involve drugs or surgery, don't expect to hear about it from your doctor! Changes to your diet and lifestyle don't just bring short term benefits; they can actually modify the genes involved in blood sugar control.

Back in the 1960s, scientists thought they understood genes pretty well. Genes were discrete bits of information that provided the blueprint for an individual person. Fixed at the moment of conception, our genetic code determined our physical characteristics and our risk of suffering from a number of inherited diseases.

Later, as more and more genes were identified, the 'nature or nurture' debate erupted, with eminent scientists unable to agree whether our genes on the one hand or our environment on the other had the greater impact on our health and development. Now, it seems that none of these ideas was quite right. The workings of the human body are infinitely more subtle and complex.

What you eat can change your genes!

Far from determining our fate, it is now clear that genes can be switched on and off by environmental factors. This means that what we eat, what pollutants we are exposed to, our daily activities and even what we experience at an emotional or social level can influence the way our genes behave. Neither our genes nor our environment is the single most important factor for our health; it is the interaction between the two that is crucial – a new field of science called epigenetics.

More startling still is the discovery that changes to the way a gene is expressed in one generation can persist and can even be carried through to the next generation. This cuts right across the long-held belief that genetic coding is set in stone and can only be changed by a random mutation in the DNA.

What relevance does this have for people with diabetes or metabolic syndrome? Plenty, as it turns out. What it means is that, even if both your parents had diabetes, what you do in terms of nutrition and lifestyle can still make a huge difference to your risk of developing the disease or the way that it progresses if you already have it *(Diabetes. 2009; 58 (12): 2718-2725)*.

Your diet, exercise and lifestyle choices don't just affect the way your body responds right now. These factors can activate or silence relevant genes, with long-term consequences for your health. For instance, experiments with mice have shown that including fish oils in the diet can activate a gene called PPARγ, which regulates insulin sensitivity and blood sugar levels *(J Nutr Biochem. 2011; 22 (2): 179-186)*.

Another epigenetic star is resveratrol, a compound found in the skins of dark grapes, which can switch on a gene called SIRT1. This has been dubbed the 'longevity gene', since it has a number of functions that protect against diabetes, heart disease and Alzheimer's disease. By activating SIRT1, resveratrol mimics the beneficial effects of a very low calorie diet (*Cell Metab. 2012; 15 (5): 675-690*).

Dietary factors are not the only things that can switch genes on or off in this way. Exercise can do it, too. A single bout of vigorous aerobic exercise activates the same PPARy gene as does fish oil for about 24 hours, improving insulin sensitivity, reducing inflammation and improving the ratio of 'good' to 'bad' cholesterol. Regular exercise over a period of several weeks means that this beneficial gene becomes permanently switched on (*J Appl Physiol. 2012; 112 (5): 806-815*).

Of course, epigenetics can also have a downside, too. One paradox of diabetes is that patients may still suffer from complications such as kidney damage or heart disease, even if their blood sugar is well-controlled. It has been suggested that even a brief exposure to high blood sugar levels may cause long-lasting changes in the way some genes are expressed, a phenomenon that has been called 'metabolic memory' (*Diabetes Technol Ther. 2012; 14 Suppl 1: S68-74*). This can mean that some harmful changes in gene action persist.

Environmental toxins can cause diabetes

Environmental toxins can also modify gene expression in ways that cause or worsen diabetes, according to two new studies presented to the Endocrine Society Annual Meeting in June 2012. Cigarette smoke is known to have gene-altering effects and now passive smoking has been linked with the development of type 2 diabetes and obesity (*Endocrine Society 94th Annual Meeting. Houston, Texas. 23-26 June 2012*).

Pesticide residues can do the same kind of damage. A second study has found that an agricultural fungicide called tolylfluanid causes insulin resistance while at the same time triggering cells to store more fat (*Endocrine Society 94th Annual Meeting. Houston, Texas. 23-26 June 2012*). This is likely to be just the tip of the toxic iceberg and we can expect many more pollutants in food, water and the air we breathe to be shown to contribute to the global epidemic of diabetes and metabolic disease.

The message from these findings is that good nutrition, regular exercise and the avoidance of environmental toxins are more important than ever for people with diabetes or metabolic syndrome.

Chinese economic boom drives diabetes time bomb

We are used to thinking of diabetes as a problem of western civilisation. However, a report recently showed that Chinese children have a rate of diabetes nearly four times greater than their counterparts in the United States. This massive rise in the incidence of diabetes is matched by increases in cardiovascular risk and, according to this study, is the result of a Chinese population that is growing increasingly overweight (*Obes Rev. 2012 Jun 28. [Epub ahead of print]*).

Perhaps these findings should not come as too much of a surprise. China has experienced unprecedented economic growth in the past two decades, coupled with equally dramatic changes in the diets and physical activity levels of its people. The stereotype of the slender, hardworking Chinese peasant is rapidly vanishing, with people in both rural and urban areas now becoming unhealthily overweight.

The study surveyed 29,000 people across the country, from 1989 to 2011. The results showed that 1.9 per cent of Chinese children aged 7 to 17 now suffer from diabetes, compared with 0.5 per cent in the United States. But this is just the tip of an iceberg of metabolic disease. In addition, 11 per cent of Chinese children and 30 per cent of Chinese adults are overweight and this figure is increasing fast. Other cardiometabolic risk factors, such as pre-diabetes, high blood sugar and high levels of cholesterol, blood fats and C-reactive protein were seen in 42 per cent of children and in around 65 per cent of adults aged 18-40.

So, what has caused this new 'China syndrome', which threatens a meltdown of the country's healthcare system if it cannot be brought under control? It is simply the result of lifestyle changes that involve less exercise (everyone used to walk or cycle, but now they drive) and more of the wrong kinds of food. After centuries of a traditional diet that relied mostly on rice, vegetables, fish and chicken, people have suddenly switched to highly processed, wheat based, high carbohydrate and high fat convenience foods.

What happens when genes and environment collide

What has happened in China is a stark illustration of epigenetics, the study of the interaction between genes and the environment, as mentioned earlier. Whereas in Europe and America the change in diet and lifestyle has been more gradual, spanning centuries rather than decades, in China it has been abrupt and its effects have been devastating.

We still have thrifty genes, geared to daily physical activity and the low-calorie food intake of the hunter-gatherer or subsistence farmer. Those genes still assume we live in a world without ready meals, fast foods, sugar, wheat or dairy produce. Our genes operate for the good of our health when they interact with a diet that is rich in plant polyphenols and low in terms of glycaemic load (GL) – that is, the degree to which it raises blood sugar levels.

What is happening in China should serve as a wake-up call to the rest of the world. As governments struggle with the massive costs involved in responding to the epidemic of diabetes, they need to take some hard decisions about the way their food industries are allowed to operate. Foods that are high in sugar or have a high GL value should carry the same stark health warnings as cigarettes.

Unfortunately, given the political clout of the global food production and processing industries, it's doubtful any such measures will be adopted any time soon and, as usual, any nod in the right direction will probably be 'too little, too late'. So, it comes down to each of us to ensure that we are doing everything we can to make the diet and lifestyle choices that will help us to reduce our risk of diabetes or to manage our condition better.

Dietary tips to help ward off diabetes:

- **Sugar: Why you should remove this poison from your diet right now**

Sometimes, following the mainstream advice on diabetes could seriously damage your health. A prime example is the role of sugar in the development of type 2 diabetes. According to Diabetes UK, "Eating sugar does not cause diabetes. Diabetes is caused by a combination of genetic and environmental factors" (*http://www.diabetes.org.uk/Get_involved/Diabetes-Week/Diabetes-Week-2010/Diabetes-myths/Eating-too-much-sugar-causes-diabetes/*). The BBC Health website says: "It's important to be aware of myths about the causes of diabetes. Eating too much sugar does not cause diabetes" (*http://www.bbc.co.uk/health/physical_health/conditions/in_depth/diabetes/aboutdiabetes_causes.shtml*).

These statements are rather like saying that a fall from a high building won't kill you. It's hitting the ground that does the damage. Well, just like stepping off a roof, eating too much sugar initiates a process that ends up with a great deal of damage being done to the body. The only difference is that in this case the process takes rather longer.

Researchers at the University of California recently claimed that sugar is so harmful that it should be controlled and taxed in the same way as tobacco and alcohol (*Lustig RH, Schmidt LA, Brindis CD. Public health: The toxic truth about sugar. Nature. 2012; 482: 27–29*). They pointed out that

78

sugar induces many of the diseases associated with 'metabolic syndrome', including high blood pressure, diabetes and accelerated ageing. In fact, they rated sugar as more dangerous to health than saturated fat and salt, which they called 'dietary bogeymen'.

In 2010, a report from the Harvard School of Public Health and Brigham and Women's Hospital, two of the most respected research institutions in the United States, concluded that: "Higher consumption of sugar sweetened beverages is associated with the development of metabolic syndrome and type 2 diabetes" (*Diabetes Care. 2010; 33(11): 2477-2483*). This finding was based on a meta-analysis of studies involving more than 300,000 patients.

A placebo-controlled, crossover clinical trial, carried out recently at the University of Zurich, Switzerland, showed that drinking low to moderate amounts of sugary drinks for just three weeks disrupted glucose and lipid metabolism and promoted inflammation in healthy young men, in ways that could lead to type 2 diabetes (*Am J Clin Nutr. 2011; 94(2): 479-485*). Even more worrying is evidence that fructose, the main sugar in sweetened soft drinks, alters the way developing fat cells in children's bodies behave, leading to insulin resistance and abdominal obesity, both of which can contribute to metabolic syndrome and type 2 diabetes (*Coade G. Fructose sugar makes maturing human fat cells fatter, less insulin-sensitive. Presentation to The Endocrine Society's 92nd Annual Meeting, San Diego, June 2010 by lead author Georgina Coade, a PhD student at the University of Bristol in the UK*).

Why is sugar so damaging to us and why are so many of us hooked on it?

The fact is that humans were never designed to eat the quantities of sugar we are exposed to today. For our hunter-gatherer ancestors, a find of wild honey was a rare treat and sweet fruits and berries were seasonal and sparse. Stone Age diets were mostly composed of fibre, protein and fats. There is just no place in our 'genetic blueprint' for large amounts of sugar and our bodies cannot cope with its sustained consumption. Refined sugar has certainly earned its popular nickname – 'the white death'. Slowly but surely, it is poisoning us.

A diet high in sugar is a sure way to raise sugar levels in the blood. High blood sugar slowly erodes the ability of cells in the pancreas to make insulin and the damage becomes permanent with time. High blood sugar also promotes the production of 'glycated proteins', which are proteins that have been damaged by binding with sugar. These glycated proteins react with oxygen to form superoxide free radicals that can degrade collagen, the structural matrix of our body, and are particularly damaging to the blood vessels.

High sugar levels and damaged blood vessels lead to the multitude of complications that can come with diabetes, including:

- Kidney disease or kidney failure

- Strokes and heart attacks

- Visual loss or blindness

- Immune system suppression

- Erectile dysfunction

- diabetic neuropathy (nerve damage)

- Poor circulation and poor wound healing

The paradox is that we are born with an attraction to sweetness, the evolutionary explanation being that sweet-tasting plants are generally safe to eat, while bitter ones may contain toxins. For some of us at least, this attraction can become an addiction. Sugar triggers the release of endorphins and dopamine, the brain's pleasure chemicals, in precisely the same way as cocaine. Sugar addiction involves the same neural receptors, neurotransmitters, and 'pleasure centres' in the brain as drug addiction and has the same symptoms of craving, dependence and withdrawal (*Psychoactive Drugs. 2010 Jun;42(2):147-51*). The more sugar we eat every day, the more hooked on it we become.

In one recent study, French researchers were amazed when they found that rats preferred water sweetened with saccharine or sugar, at about the concentrations found in soft drinks, to hits of cocaine – exactly the opposite of what had been predicted. "It was a big surprise," explained Serge Ahmed, a neuroscientist who led the research at the University of Bordeaux (*PLoS One. 2010; 5(2): e9296*).

Luckily, this is one addiction that you can break relatively easily and your body will thank you for doing so. The main thing is to be aware of everything you put into your mouth and follow a low-GL way of eating. A diet that includes plenty of good quality protein, fish oils, nuts and seeds and fresh green vegetables will help to cut sugar cravings. Say no to desserts and switch to water or herbal tea instead of soft drinks. Once you get through the first few days, you are likely to be amazed at how quickly your sweet cravings disappear as you cut out sugar and simple carbohydrates and keep your blood sugar in balance.

• Artificial sweeteners can affect blood sugar control

Because eating sugar (sucrose) is a sure route to weight gain, many people use artificial sweeteners as an alternative. People with diabetes are often advised to use these products as an aid to keeping their blood sugar levels stable. But how much do we know about artificial sweeteners and the effects they may be having on our body processes?

It has been recognised for some time that, as the use of artificial sweeteners has grown worldwide, the incidence of obesity has been rising in parallel. Scientists have started asking whether these sweeteners, far from helping people to lose weight, are actually contributing to weight gain. The answer, it seems, lies in the way our brains respond to sugar, which, as mentioned previously, is an addictive substance that triggers the brain's reward centres in just the same way as drugs such as cocaine and morphine. But when sweetness is provided without accompanying calories, this addiction is not fully satisfied. Instead, artificial sweeteners encourage greater sugar cravings and sugar dependence (*Yale J Biol Med. 2010; 83 (2): 101-108*).

So, while you may feel virtuous using a sweetener instead of sugar in your tea or coffee, doing so can fuel an on-going need to reach for something sweet. Using sweeteners as part of a weight loss plan could actually make it more difficult to stick to a healthy diet and, in the end, contribute to weight gain.

It's important to point out that there are big differences between artificial sweeteners. Some have been associated with effects that are detrimental to health, while others have been found to be quite beneficial. Heading the list of 'villains' is aspartame (Nutra Sweet), over which controversy has raged for some years. It has been linked to brain and nerve diseases, such as multiple sclerosis, dementia, epilepsy and Parkinson's disease.

Aspartame and xylitol have opposite effects on insulin sensitivity

Especially relevant for people with diabetes or metabolic syndrome are the results of new research showing that aspartame can reduce insulin sensitivity, in mice at least. Compared to controls, mice fed aspartame long-term had higher fasting blood glucose levels and showed a greater degree of insulin resistance (*PLoS One. 2012; 7 (4): e31570*). The aspartame-fed mice also took longer to learn how to escape from a maze and made more mistakes, suggesting that aspartame may also affect memory and spatial awareness. In a separate new study, aspartame was found to cause free radical damage in the brains of rats, due to its conversion to methanol, a brain toxin (*J Biosci. 2012; 37 (4): 679-688*).

Leading for the 'heroes' is a sweetener called xylitol, which newly published research has shown to prevent the development of insulin resistance in rats (*Diabetologia. 2012; 55 (6): 1808-1812*). The animals were given direct infusions of lipids to raise their blood fat levels, which resulted in a 25 per cent reduction in insulin sensitivity. However, this drop in insulin sensitivity was prevented if xylitol was infused into the rats' blood at the same time. Although this effect needs to be tested in humans consuming xylitol as a sweetener, the results hold considerable promise for diabetes sufferers.

Another sweetener that may help to stabilise blood sugar is a natural herb called stevia. When rats were treated with alloxan, a chemical that causes damage to the insulin-producing cells in the pancreas, their blood sugar levels rose; but if they were then given stevia for 10 days, normal blood sugar levels were restored (*J Pharm Bioallied Sci. 201; 3 (2): 242-248*). Compared with the anti-diabetes drug glibenclamide, stevia normalised blood sugar safely, without the swing to hypoglycaemia (dangerously low blood sugar) associated with the drug. In a separate study, the main active chemical in stevia (rebauside A) was again shown to reduce blood sugar levels in diabetic rats (*J Physiol Biochem. 2012; 68 (3): 421-431*).

It probably makes the most sense to try and reduce your intake of both sugar and artificial sweeteners as far as possible, in order to control the feeling that you need to eat something sweet. If you want to continue to use a sugar alternative, it seems that aspartame is definitely best avoided while xylitol or stevia could be beneficial in helping with blood sugar control.

• The impact of saturated fats and omega-3 fatty acids on type 2 diabetes

For the last thirty years, we have been hearing the low fat message: dietary fat leads to weight gain, high cholesterol levels and heart disease. More recently, the finger has been pointed specifically at saturated fats, the kind you find in butter and lamb chops, for instance, as being the villains of the piece. So, what is the real truth about fats and how do they fit into the diabetes picture?

Fats, including the saturated kind, are essential elements of our diet and have multiple functions in our bodies. Among other things, they are used to construct cell membranes and nerve sheaths and they form the raw materials from which we manufacture sex hormones, vitamin D and countless other important substances. In 2009, a systematic review of studies investigating a causal link between dietary factors and coronary heart disease concluded that there was no evidence to support an overall reduction of saturated fatty acids in the diet (*Arch Intern Med 2009; 169 (7): 659–669*).

Saturated fats block glucose uptake in pancreatic beta cells

That said, recent research has shed light on a way in which saturated fats may be implicated in the development of diabetes. In healthy people, beta cells in the pancreas constantly monitor the bloodstream for glucose. When blood sugar is high, beta cells take in glucose, through glucose transporters in their cell membranes, and respond by secreting insulin in a timed and measured way. In turn, insulin then stimulates other cells in the body to take up glucose. Animal studies at the University of California have discovered that high fat diets and consequent high levels of blood fats interfere with a process that maintains the glucose transport mechanism in pancreatic beta cells (*Nat Med 2011; 17 (9): 1067-1075*). So, when the researchers fed otherwise normal mice a diet high in saturated fats, they found that the animals' beta cells could no longer sense and respond to blood glucose.

That research suggests that we should be avoiding too much fat in our diets if we want to prevent type 2 diabetes or limit its effects. But the evidence on this is not clear cut, since another recent study found that higher intakes of dietary fibre, but not low intakes of saturated fat or cholesterol, reduced the risk of metabolic syndrome in American teenagers (*J Am Diet Assoc 2011; 111 (11): 1688-1695*). These findings point to the inclusion of fibre-rich, nutrient-dense, plant-based foods as being more important than restricting total fat, cholesterol, or saturated fat intake, for maintaining insulin sensitivity and good blood sugar control.

Omega-3 fats could prevent type 2 diabetes and its cardiac complications

While saturated fats may or may not be involved in the development of type 2 diabetes, there is plenty of evidence on the beneficial effects of polyunsaturated fats, particularly the omega-3 fatty acids found in fish and some seed oils. Two recent studies on Chinese populations have confirmed that omega-3 fatty acid intake is associated with a reduced risk of type 2 diabetes. However, while one of these found that eating seafood had benefits (*Am J Clin Nutr 2011; 94 (2): 543-551*), the other concluded that only plant-derived omega-3 fats had this effect (*Am J Clin Nutr 2011; 94(2):520-526*). A further study, from the US, found that both marine and plant sourced omega-3 fatty acids were linked with a lower risk of diabetes, but in this instance the association was with levels in the blood of study participants, rather than with their dietary intakes (*Am J Clin Nutr 2011; 94 (2): 527-533*).

The contradictory conclusions arrived at by these two Chinese population studies may simply reflect the fact that we are all different. This was demonstrated by a new Spanish study, which found an association between blood levels of specific fatty acids and insulin receptor functions in people with one variant of a particular gene, but not in those having a different variant (*Mol Nutr Food Res 2011. [Epub ahead of print]*).

For people who are already living with diabetes, omega-3 fatty acids may help to reduce the risk of complications. A Dutch research team has found that people aged 60 to 80 and suffering from diabetes, who took a relatively small supplement of omega-3s, had a significantly lower risk of a fatal heart attack or arrhythmia event than those taking placebo (*Diabetes Care. 2011; 34 (12): 2515-2520*). In this trial, participants used margarines containing eicosapentaenoic acid (EPA), docosahexaenoic acid (DHA) or alpha-linolenic acid (ALA).

The message from these studies is twofold. First, it may be advisable to limit your intake of saturated fats, since they could interfere with your body's normal response to elevated blood sugar and so could contribute to the development of type 2 diabetes. Second, making sure that you get plenty of omega-3 fatty acids, from oily fish, hemp seeds, linseeds and walnuts could reduce your risk of developing type 2 diabetes and your risk of cardiovascular disease.

- ### Eating pulses improves blood sugar control in diabetes

People following a low carbohydrate diet often view with suspicion pulses such as lentils, kidney beans and chickpeas. It is true that, with the exception of soya (edamame) beans, these are all 'starchy' foods that have a moderately high carbohydrate content. However, a new study has found that eating more of them, as part of a low GL diet, improves blood sugar control and reduces the risk of coronary heart disease, in people with type 2 diabetes (*Arch Intern Med. 2012 Oct 22 [Epub ahead of print]*).

The research, carried out in Toronto, Canada, involved 121 type 2 diabetes patients. They were already following a low GL diet and this was supplemented with either additional pulses or additional whole wheat products, over the course of three months. Changes in their haemoglobin A1c (HbA1c) values, an indicator of long-term blood sugar control, were recorded and coronary heart disease risk scores were also calculated for each patient.

It has to be said that the changes in HbA1c values were very modest; down by 0.5 per cent for those eating additional pulses and by 0.3 per cent for the group getting additional wheat products. The bean eaters also saw an average drop of 4.5 points in their systolic blood pressure, which led to a 0.8 per cent reduction in their heart disease risk. Although these beneficial effects were small, they show that pulses are a valuable component of the diet for anybody with diabetes. And it is likely that a longer study period would have shown greater effects.

In fact, an earlier, long-term analysis of food intake patterns and death risk from coronary heart disease has revealed that pulses have a much more substantial effect than the new study suggests. When researchers monitored more than 16,000 middle-aged men in the US, Japan and Europe for 25 years, they found that those eating the most pulses had a massive 82 per cent reduction in death risk (*Eur J Epidemiol 1999; 15 (6): 507-515*).

In countries where pulses are a staple part of the diet, diabetes rates tend to be low. The typical western diet, on the other hand, doesn't contain enough of these nutritious foods. The only one we consume much of is tinned baked beans, which usually come with a large dose of added sugar. Eating pulses has been associated with a reduced risk of type 2 diabetes and some studies have also shown that they improve glucose tolerance. Pulses have been found to lower postprandial (after meal) glucose and insulin responses, a benefit that applies not only to the meal at which they were eaten but also the subsequent meal four hours later – or even until breakfast the next day if they are eaten in the evening.

Pulses slow down starch digestion and sugar release

Just by including pulses in a meal, you will reduce the GL of that meal. Pulses are an excellent source of soluble fibre, which slows down the release of sugars from foods in the gut, delaying their absorption so that their impact on blood sugar is reduced. Compounds in soluble fibre also help to control blood sugar by inhibiting the action of the enzymes that digest starch. Lentils, in particular, may have yet another trick up their sleeve. They are one of the best natural sources of the trace element molybdenum, which has been shown in laboratory tests to improve insulin sensitivity and to increase the secretion of insulin from pancreatic beta-cells (*Biol Trace Elem Res. 2010; 133 (2): 236-241*).

While all pulses are good for controlling blood sugar levels, some are better than others. Those with the lowest glycaemic load (GL), which have the least effect on blood sugar, are Borlotti beans and lentils, followed by butter beans, kidney beans and chickpeas. In fact, you could eat double the portion of Borlotti beans compared with chickpeas and get the same blood sugar response. Lentils are easier than the other kinds of pulses to cook, since they do not require soaking beforehand. Alternatively, many kinds of pulses are available ready cooked and tinned – just check that they have no added sugar.

• How dietary fibre could help control type 2 diabetes

In the 1970s, science started to reveal the value of 'dietary fibre' not only for preventing constipation but also for reducing cholesterol and lowering the risk of bowel cancer and other diseases.

Today, a clear link has been established between fibre intake and the control of type 2 diabetes. In early 2012 scientists at the Medical University of South Carolina in the US carried out a meta-analysis of the results of 15 separate clinical trials in which additional dietary fibre was given to people with type 2 diabetes (*J Am Board Fam Med. 2012; 25 (1): 16-23*). They concluded that providing a dietary fibre supplement to these patients caused significant falls in both fasting blood sugar and glycosylated haemoglobin (HbA1c) levels.

If you have diabetes, you will be familiar with both of these readings. Fasting blood sugar is a direct measurement of the level of glucose in your blood after an overnight fast and it shows just how effective insulin is at removing glucose from your bloodstream at the time of the test. Glycosylated haemoglobin is a compound formed by the interaction of glucose with haemoglobin in the blood and its level provides a reliable indication of how good your blood sugar control is over the longer term.

So, what is dietary fibre and how does it affect blood sugar levels? Generally speaking, dietary fibre is that part of plant foods that is resistant to digestion and absorption in the small intestine. In other words, it's what goes straight through us. It is split into two main categories, insoluble fibre and soluble fibre. Insoluble fibre includes the things that come to mind for most of us when we think of fibre – wheat bran, the skins of fruits and vegetables, celery, salads and so forth. It provides bulk in the intestine, speeds up transit time and absorbs water to make the stools softer.

When is a fibre not a fibre?

Soluble fibre is a bit of a misnomer as it isn't really fibrous. It includes gums and mucilages that dissolve to become gelatinous and sticky liquids that are fermented by the gut bacteria. This category of fibre includes prebiotics that are used to encourage the growth of friendly bacteria, as well as substances such as beta-glucans that have been shown to support the immune system.

Foods that are high in fibre tend to have low GL (glycaemic load) scores, a measure of how they affect blood sugar levels. Soluble fibre, in particular, helps to slow down the release of sugars from foods in the gut and to delay their absorption, which means that their impact on blood sugar is reduced.

Another recent meta-analysis of clinical trials found that a type of soluble fibre called fructo-oligosaccharide (FOS), which is also a popular prebiotic, had a beneficial influence on glucose metabolism, with one study showing a marked reduction in blood sugar levels in people with type 2 diabetes, after taking eight grams of FOS a day for two weeks (*Acta Cir Bras. 2012; 27 (3): 279-282*).

The second way in which soluble fibre compounds help to control blood sugar is by inhibiting the action of the enzymes that digest starch (*Mini Rev Med Chem. 2010; 10 (4): 315-331*). This means that the carbohydrate in, say, potatoes or white rice is converted to sugar much more slowly because the enzyme that catalyses the conversion works less well. The result is less of a spike in blood sugar levels when you eat these foods.

Dietary fibre could reduce inflammation and fat deposition

Research carried out at University College Medical School in London has suggested yet another mechanism through which dietary fibre can aid blood sugar control (*Diabetes Care. 2009; 32 (10): 1823-1825*). In this study, 3,428 non-diabetic men were monitored for seven years, during which time 162 of them developed type 2 diabetes. Analysis of their diets found that those eating the least fibre had the highest risk of diabetes and blood tests showed that low fibre intake also correlated with increased inflammatory markers and fat deposition in the liver – inflammation and visceral fat are directly connected with the development of insulin resistance and type 2 diabetes.

Some of the best sources of soluble fibre are oats, barley, beans, lentils, apples and citrus fruits. Linseeds and chia seeds (from a Mexican plant related to sage) are particularly high in soluble fibre and make a good addition to muesli, porridge or salads. You could also use one of the many soluble fibre supplements on the market, such as psyllium, apple pectin, FOS or glucomannan.

Making even small dietary and lifestyle changes can make a big difference

To demonstrate how significant even a small reduction of glucose can be, consider the Diabetes Control and Complications Trial in the US, which was conducted from 1983 to 1993 by the National Institute of Diabetes and Digestive and Kidney Diseases (NIDDK). The researchers found that even a 2 per cent decrease in blood glucose levels produced dramatic results: a 75 per cent reduced risk of developing eye problems, a 50 per cent reduced risk of kidney disease, and a 60 per cent reduced risk of developing a nerve disorder (*N Engl J Med 1993; 329: 997-986*).

• Can cheese cut your diabetes risk?

Some national newspapers recently ran a story, based on the results of a new study, which suggested that eating cheese could reduce the risk of developing type 2 diabetes. But before you rush out to stock up your fridge, let's take a look at what the study really found and how cheese and other dairy produce might affect diabetes.

The study in question used Europe-wide data on eating habits and health to compare the dairy product intakes of over 12,000 people who developed type 2 diabetes with a random sample of others who did not (*Am J Clin Nutr. 2012; 96 (2): 382-390*). It concluded that overall, there was no association between total dairy product intake and the risk of developing type 2 diabetes.

People who ate the most fermented dairy products, which included yoghurt, other kinds of fermented milk and cheese, had a 12 per cent reduced risk of developing diabetes. However, when researchers looked at these foods individually, there were no clear associations.

In fact, the difference in risk varied widely from country to country; people in France who ate more cheese had a reduced risk of developing diabetes, while those in the UK who ate more cheese were actually at increased risk! The researchers did not examine the types of cheese eaten, which could have affected the results. For instance, in France, much of the cheese is made from goat's milk or ewe's milk, rather than cow's milk.

So, the idea that eating an extra two slices of cheese a day could prevent diabetes, as suggested by some newspapers, may be misleading. The study did suggest that there may be some benefit from fermented dairy products in general, which merited further investigation and the authors speculated that this could be due to the types of fats or the probiotic bacteria contained in these products; but those things were not examined in this study.

Studies show inconsistent results on the link between dairy and diabetes

Another three studies have recently been published on the same subject. A study carried out in Australia, contrary to the European findings, concluded that total dairy intake was associated with a lower risk of diabetes, in men at least (*Public Health Nutr. 2012 Jun 7. [Epub ahead of print]*). The same trend was found to a lesser degree in women, but was not statistically significant (in other words, it could have been due to chance).

On the other hand, a study from the Netherlands, which subdivided dairy products into low-fat and high-fat, found no associations between diabetes risk and intakes of either total dairy or fermented dairy products (*Br J Nutr. 2012 Jun 7. [Epub ahead of print]*).

Finally, a comprehensive literature review from the US examined 16 separate studies and concluded that, although the results are inconsistent, overall they suggest that the consumption of high-fat dairy products is linked to a lower incidence of obesity, type 2 diabetes and cardiovascular disease (*Eur J Nutr. 2012 Jul 19. [Epub ahead of print]*). This is just the opposite of what we are usually told by mainstream medics, who advocate a low fat diet!

So what do you do? It seems that the jury is still out on the link between dairy products and diabetes. But at least there is little evidence that eating them has a detrimental effect on diabetes risk (if you ignore the finding from the Europe study about cheese intake in the UK!). From the findings, it is probably fair to assume that eating dairy foods, including cheese, in moderation, is fine. Much more important than focusing on these foods alone is to follow a low-GL diet that limits sugar and carbohydrates, which have devastating effects on your blood sugar and insulin levels.

- ## Nuts: A simple way to manage type 2 diabetes and prevent complications

According to the latest research findings, daily consumption of nuts may help to control type 2 diabetes and prevent its complications (*Diabetes Care. 2011 Aug; 34 (8): 1706-1711*).

The researchers found that consuming two ounces of nuts a day, as a replacement for carbohydrates, appears to be an effective glycaemic and serum lipid control for type 2 diabetes sufferers.

Many nuts, including cashews, walnuts, and almonds, are known to have higher levels of monounsaturated fatty acids, and have been touted as potentially having anti-diabetic effects. Nuts also contain fibre, vitamin E, omega-3 fatty acids, plant sterols, and L-argine.

The researchers noted that fat intake, especially monounsaturated fatty acids, have been shown to preserve HDL cholesterol and improve glycaemic control, in diabetic patients, "yet the exact sources have not been clearly defined," they said.

Lead researcher Dr. David Jenkins, from the University of Toronto, and his team who carried out the study, assessed the effect of mixed nut consumption on serum lipids and blood sugar control in type 2 diabetes.

The researchers divided 117 patients with type 2 diabetes into three different groups. Each group was given a different supplementary meal for a period of three months: One group was given 'healthy' muffins (so-called because the muffin was made of whole wheat products, sweetened with apple concentrate, and had no sugar added); one was provided with a mixture of two ounces of nuts including raw almonds, pistachios, walnuts, pecans, hazelnuts, peanuts, cashews, and macadamias; and one group was given a mixture of muffins and nuts.

People receiving the nut-only supplement reported the greatest improvement in blood glucose control, and were also found to have a reduction in low-density lipoprotein 'bad' (LDL) cholesterol.

The researchers found that patients given muffins and mixed muffin-and-nuts experienced no significant improvement in their blood sugar control. Those receiving the muffin-nut mixture significantly lowered their serum LDL cholesterol levels, while the muffin group showed no decrease in LDL levels.

Patients receiving the full dose of nuts reduced their HbA1c – a long-term marker of blood sugar control – by two-thirds of what the US Food and Drug Administration (FDA) recognizes as being clinically meaningful for therapeutic agents.

Commenting on the findings, Dr. David Jenkins said: "Mixed, unsalted, raw, or dry-roasted nuts have benefits for both blood glucose control and blood lipids and may be used as part of a strategy to improve diabetes control without weight gain."

"Neither in the current study nor in previous reports has nut consumption been associated with weight gain. If anything, nuts appear to be well suited as part of weight-reducing diets."

• Make fish a part of your anti-diabetes diet

Research at the University of Valencia that analysed dietary patterns in a Spanish adult population has found that fish appears to protect against the development of type 2 diabetes (*Nutr Hosp. 2011 Oct; 26 (5): 1033-1040*).

The study aimed to understand current eating patterns in terms of meat and fish consumption and the correlation between the Mediterranean diet and cardiovascular risk factors. What the researchers discovered was that the Mediterranean population they looked at ate considerable amounts of both red meat and fish. But, while the consumption of red meat, especially cured meats, was related to increased weight gain and obesity, eating fish was associated with a lower prevalence of type 2 diabetes and lower blood glucose levels.

In itself, this study only shows an association and does not prove that fish reduces diabetes risk. It is likely, though, that eating a lot of fish leads to high levels of omega-3 fatty acids in the cells of the skeletal muscles. According to a recent study at the University of Cordoba, omega-3 fatty acids in muscle cells interact with genes controlling insulin sensitivity, so helping to reduce fasting glucose levels in people with metabolic syndrome (*Mol Nutr Food Res. 2011 Dec 7. [Epub ahead of print]*).

As a general guide, aim to eat fish (oily fish – such as mackerel, sardines and salmon – if possible) three times a week.

- ## The occasional glass of red wine could help control diabetes

Research has shown that resveratrol – found most abundantly in the skins of red grapes – can help manage diabetes. Resveratrol is a natural polyphenol that plants produce to protect themselves from attack by bacteria and fungi. It has been suspected for some time of having several beneficial health properties, but was recently under a cloud due to the discovery of some falsified results from a single researcher. Regrettable as this is, it highlights the importance of only relying on studies that have been independently verified by two or more respected institutions.

Resveratrol has already shown promising effects on insulin sensitivity and glucose tolerance in several animal studies, but now these have been confirmed in the first human clinical trial (*J Gerontol A Biol Sci Med Sci. 2012 Jan 4. [Epub ahead of print]*). This was a small, pilot study with 10 people aged 69 to 75, diagnosed with impaired glucose tolerance (also called 'pre-diabetes'), who were given a moderate dose supplement of resveratrol for four weeks. The results showed significant improvements in insulin sensitivity and reduced post-meal glucose levels.

The way that resveratrol appears to work in the body is by inhibiting certain enzymes known as phosphodiesterases, that help regulate cell energy. In mice, at least, this has the effect of preventing diet-induced obesity, improving glucose tolerance and increasing physical endurance. To get more resveratrol into your diet, red grapes and red wine (drunk in moderation… such as a glass of red wine three or four days a week) are the best sources. It is also present in raisins, blueberries, raspberries, peanuts and pistachios.

- ## Pumpkins can help you avoid or better manage diabetes

A portion of pumpkin has a low glycaemic load (GL), about one sixth of that of a baked potato.

The vibrant orange colour of pumpkins comes from beta-carotene, a plant pigment that is also a fat-soluble antioxidant and is converted to vitamin A in the body. Animal studies have suggested that beta-carotene helps to protect against diseases in which oxidative processes play a role, such as the complications that can arise from diabetes. Reactive oxygen species (free radicals) are produced by the immune system as a natural defence against invading pathogens, but when they are present in excess they can cause vascular complications in diabetes.

A recent study from Brazil showed that diabetic rats produced significantly more reactive oxygen species than non-diabetic controls (*J Clin Biochem Nutr. 2012; 50 (3): 177-183*). Including beta-carotene in the feed of diabetic rats was found to reduce the levels of reactive oxygen species present, indicating that it may help to prevent conditions linked to oxidative stress, such as heart disease, diabetic retinopathy and diabetic nephropathy.

Beta-carotene is not the only diabetes-fighting nutrient in pumpkins. Two other compounds, trigonelline and nicotinic acid, have been shown in studies to be effective in lowering blood sugar levels by improving insulin resistance. Researchers in Japan used non-obese, type 2 diabetic rats, as a model for the condition in humans. They found that when pumpkin was added to the feed of one group of these rats, their blood sugar levels remained lower than those of a control group, during a glucose tolerance test (*Biosci Biotechnol Biochem. 2009; 73 (5): 1033-1041*).

Pumpkin compounds have multiple modes of action against diabetes

This study went on to isolate the two compounds responsible for the blood sugar lowering effect and found that trigonelline and nicotinic acid both improved glucose tolerance, with a stronger effect from trigonelline. This is not surprising, since trigonelline is the active compound in fenugreek (*Trigonella foenum-graecum*), a herb with a long tradition of use in India for the treatment of diabetes. Trigonelline acts by supporting the regeneration of beta-cells (the insulin-producing cells in the pancreas), increasing insulin secretion and regulating the activity of enzymes related to glucose metabolism, as well as acting as an antioxidant (*Curr Med Chem. 2012; 19 (21): 3523-3531*).

Other members of the squash family also have beneficial effects on blood sugar levels. In Mexico, researchers have found that a kind of pumpkin called the fig-leaf gourd contains the phytochemical D-chiro-inositol, which has blood sugar lowering properties comparable to standard anti-diabetic drugs and is also an antioxidant and anti-inflammatory (*Am J Chin Med. 2012; 40 (1): 97-110*). The bitter melon, another kind of gourd grown widely in Asia, Africa and the Caribbean, has been found to improve insulin sensitivity, increase insulin production, reduce blood sugar levels, suppress appetite and repair damaged beta-cells in the pancreas (*J Med Food. 2012; 15 (2): 101-107*).

Pumpkins can be eaten roasted, baked or steamed as a side vegetable and are great added to risotto or curry or made into a warming winter soup. And don't forget to eat the pumpkin seeds, too, which are best lightly roasted. The polyunsaturated fatty acids in pumpkin seed oil play a vital role in skin health, promoting its natural moisture balance and lubrication, and also help to prevent menopausal symptoms in women and benign enlargement of the prostate gland in men.

• **Diabetes benefits linked to strawberries**

Recent scientific studies have revealed that compounds in strawberries (a low glycaemic index food) may reduce the risks of diabetic complications. Strawberries contain health-promoting compounds known as flavonoids, including a particular one called fisetin. In fact, strawberries are the richest natural source of fisetin.

What makes fisetin special is its potential to reverse some diabetic complications. Scientists at the Salk Institute for Biological Studies, in California, studied the effects of fisetin in Akita mice, which have increased blood sugar typical of type 1 diabetes and show the pathologies typical of serious diabetic complications in humans (*PLoS One. 2011; 6 (6): e21226*).

These include diabetic nephropathy or kidney disease, retinopathy, and neuropathies, in which patients lose touch or heat sensations.

Mice fed a fisetin-enriched diet remained diabetic, but acute kidney enlargement was reversed, and high urine protein levels, a sure indication of kidney disease, fell. In addition, blood and brain levels of sugars attached to proteins, known as advanced glycation end-products or AGEs, were reduced in fisetin-treated mice. High levels of AGEs have been linked with most of the complications of diabetes.

What is true for mice may not always apply to humans, so it is good to see that in a recent clinical trial strawberries also reduced risk factors for cardiovascular disease, stroke and diabetes in obese people (*Br J Nutr. 2011 Nov 9:1-10. [Epub ahead of print]*). In this study, 20 subjects with a body mass index (BMI) between 30 and 40 were given either dried strawberry powder or a strawberry-flavoured placebo for three weeks.

The groups were then swapped around for a further three weeks in what is known as a crossover trial. Blood tests showed that strawberry powder reduced levels of cholesterol and small HDL ('good') cholesterol particles, and increased LDL ('bad') particle size in obese subjects. The latest thinking is that cholesterol particle size is a more reliable indicator of cardiovascular risk than either HDL or LDL cholesterol levels. When LDL particles are small, a heightened risk of cardiovascular disease remains even if overall LDL counts are at ideal levels.

•   **Forget 'diabetic chocolate' and try the real McCoy**

When it comes to chocolate, people with diabetes have long been told to avoid it, because of its high sugar and fat content. So-called 'diabetic chocolate' is little better, often containing unhealthy artificial sweeteners and trans-fats. In the last few years though, research has revealed that dark chocolate, which is relatively low in sugar, has considerable health benefits.

In a series of clinical trials, researchers at L'Aquila University in Italy discovered that dark chocolate, which is rich in compounds called flavanols, improved insulin sensitivity and pancreatic beta-cell function, reduced blood pressure and improved blood vessel dilation in people with high blood pressure and insulin resistance (*J Nutr. 2008; 138 (9): 1671-1676*).

Another study at the University of Hull, in the UK, found that dark chocolate increased levels of HDL ('good') cholesterol in people with type 2 diabetes (*Diabet Med. 2010; 27 (11): 1318-1321*). A scientific review of the health benefits of dark chocolate confirmed its powerful antioxidant and anti-inflammatory activity and its ability to improve insulin sensitivity and reduce the risk of type 2 diabetes (*Antioxid Redox Signal. 2011; 15 (10): 2779-2811*).

The darker the chocolate, the higher its concentration of beneficial flavanols and the lower its sugar content, so try to go for one that has at least 70 per cent cocoa solids. Once you are used to this, you can graduate to the 85 or 90 per cent stuff! There's a bit of an art to eating this kind of chocolate – rather than chewing it, just break off a small piece and let it melt on your tongue. That way, you'll really appreciate its wonderful flavour and texture.

• **Add these magnesium-rich foods to your shopping list to ward off type 2 diabetes**

To prevent type 2 diabetes get out your shopping list and add these items: leafy green vegetables, avocados, nuts and whole grains. Each of these foods is high in magnesium – a nutrient that, according to the results of a new study, may be a key player in preventing type 2 diabetes.

Before looking at this important new finding in more detail, here's what researchers have already discovered about magnesium and metabolic syndrome – a set of symptoms including excessive abdominal fat, elevated triglyceride and CRP levels, low HDL (the 'good' form of cholesterol), high blood pressure, and a fasting glucose level that would indicate possible insulin resistance... Three or more of these symptoms are all that's required to diagnose metabolic syndrome. In the US, surveys estimate that as many as one in four adults has metabolic syndrome, which increases the risk of diabetes and cardiovascular disease, and UK research suggests a similar number of people are affected here.

In 2005, researchers from Brigham and Women's Hospital collected dietary and medical data from more than 11,000 women over the age of 45 who participated in the on-going Women's Health Study. Results showed that subjects with the highest magnesium intake had a 27 per cent lower risk of developing metabolic syndrome (*Diabetes Care, Vol. 28, No. 6, June 2005*).

The following year, Northwestern University researchers reported on a study in which dietary and medical records for more than 4,600 healthy subjects were followed for 15 years. As in the Brigham and Women's study, the highest intake of magnesium was linked with a significantly lower risk of metabolic syndrome.

These results are not entirely surprising. Previous research suggests that magnesium helps heart muscles relax, reduces blood pressure, and helps control homocysteine and C-reactive protein levels.

Lower your risk of diabetes through magnesium supplements or dietary measures alone

The latest magnesium/diabetes research comes from the Karolinska Institute in Stockholm, Sweden. The Karolinska team reviewed seven large studies similar to the two above – in each study, dietary and medical records were followed over a long period.

Four studies tracked diet only, while three studies reviewed dietary habits and supplement intake. The combined studies included more than 286,000 subjects.

Results: Six of the studies found a significant association between high magnesium intake and a reduced risk of type 2 diabetes. The sources of magnesium – whether from diet or supplements combined with diet – were equally effective. Diabetes risk dropped by 15 per cent for every 100mg increase in magnesium intake (*Journal of Internal Medicine, Vol. 262, No. 2, August 2007*).

Other health benefits associated with magnesium include the promotion of bone health in postmenopausal women and a reduced risk of cognitive decline (*Endocrinol Metab Clin N Am 1998, 27(2) 389-398*).

Could you be suffering from a magnesium deficiency?

Unfortunately, it's quite easy to become magnesium deficient. High stress and menstruation can take their toll on magnesium levels, while a heavy intake of starches, alcohol, diuretics and some prescription drugs (such as antibiotics) can increase urinary excretion of magnesium.

If a blood test shows your magnesium level is low (a normal range is anywhere between 0.66 and 1.23 millimoles per litre), you can help make up this shortfall by taking 500mg of magnesium per day. Magnesium gluconate and chelated magnesium are the preferred supplement forms. As always, talk to your doctor before adding magnesium to your supplement regimen.

•   Eat a high-antioxidant diet

Research has revealed that oxidative stress appears to play a major role in the development of diabetes.

Normal biological functions naturally produce highly reactive molecules called free radicals, also called 'reactive oxygen species'. These molecules have toxic or damaging effects in the body, which are counteracted by antioxidants that the body produces or that are present in foods.

There is a constant war going on between free radicals and antioxidants. When there is insufficient antioxidant capacity to balance out the effects of free radicals, the result is oxidative stress. Many scientists now believe that almost all of the disease processes in the body involve oxidative stress as a 'final common pathway' (*Rev Diabet Stud. 2010; 7 (1): 15-25*).

In diabetes, oxidative stress is involved in three main ways: damaging the insulin-producing beta-cells in the pancreas; contributing to insulin resistance; and causing changes to blood vessels that result in diabetic complications (heart disease, kidney damage and eye problems). It is also involved in obesity and high blood pressure, two conditions that frequently accompany diabetes (*Clin Chem Lab Med. 2011; 49 (11): 1773-1782*).

High levels of blood sugar and blood fats cause oxidative stress in the pancreatic beta-cells, which produce insulin. The beta-cells are especially vulnerable to this kind of damage, which results in lowered output of insulin and increased cell death (*Pflugers Arch. 2010; 460 (4): 703-718*). This means that the pancreas cannot always produce sufficient insulin to deal with the level of sugar in the blood, leading to chronic high sugar levels which are in turn a cause of further oxidative stress. In this way a 'vicious cycle' of damage to the pancreas is set up.

To help counteract the damaging effects of oxidative stress, you should make sure your diet contains plenty of antioxidant-rich foods. These include:

- Blueberries, cherries, raspberries and other 'summer fruits';

- Broccoli, kale, red cabbage and garlic;

- Kidney beans, lentils and chick peas;

- Walnuts, pecans and pistachio nuts;

- Apples, pears, oranges, grapefruit and plums;

- Dark chocolate (70 per cent cocoa solids or higher);

- Coffee, black and green tea;

- Red wine (in moderation!).

• The hidden ingredient in soft drinks that increases diabetes risk

There are plenty of good reasons to avoid fructose, but all you need is one: Type 2 diabetes.

A new study highlights diabetes and all the other key reasons why it's essential to avoid this dangerous component of processed foods and soft drinks.

The research findings speak for themselves...

An animal study carried out in 2002 by US researchers at the University of California, Davis (UCD) showed how fructose consumption contributed to insulin resistance, high blood pressure, and elevated triglyceride levels – three of the core symptoms of metabolic syndrome which put a patient at high risk of developing type 2 diabetes and heart disease. In the conclusions to their 2002 study, the UCD team noted that a high intake of fructose might increase body weight and encourage insulin resistance.

Then, in 2007, the same UCD researchers conducted a human study, the results of which they presented at the American Diabetes Association 67th Annual Scientific Sessions in Chicago, which confirmed these results. They began by giving a series of tests to assess heart disease risk in 23 overweight adults, aged 43 to 70.

Study profile:

- For two weeks, each subject ate a strict diet that consisted of 30 per cent fat, and 55 per cent complex carbohydrates.

- After the first phase was complete, subjects were allowed to eat whatever they liked for eight weeks, along with three sweetened beverages each day that supplied a quarter of their energy intake – about half the group drank a glucose beverage while the other half drank a fructose beverage.

- After the second phase was complete, subjects returned to the 30/55 diet while continuing with their daily drinks.

- Throughout the study, further checks of heart disease indicators occurred at two, eight, and 10 weeks.

Results showed that just two weeks after subjects began drinking sweetened drinks, triglyceride levels were up in the fructose group, but had actually dropped in the glucose group.

Over the entire range of the study, LDL cholesterol increased and insulin sensitivity decreased in the fructose group but didn't change in the glucose group. In addition, fructose subjects gained about three pounds overall, but no weight gain was reported in the glucose group.

A fructose by any other name...

UCD researcher, Dr Peter J. Havel (who participated in both the 2002 and 2007 studies), told WebMD Medical News that most people get added sugars in their diet from daily beverages – which tends to be a lifelong habit, far exceeding the two weeks in which fructose quickly had an adverse effect on triglycerides.

So what exactly is in that vast array of choices in the beverage aisle?

Checking the ingredients of your soft drink, sports tea, vitamin water, power drink, etc., you might wonder what the difference is between fructose, high fructose corn syrup (HFCS), and crystalline fructose. Is one better than the other? Well... put it this way: If only part of your house is on fire, your house is still on fire.

The average high fructose corn syrup is made up of about 50 per cent fructose.

But according to the Sugar Association (sugar.org), increased fructose content of HFCS is becoming more common. Some of these syrups contain more than 90 per cent fructose.

And then there's crystalline fructose that's present in many 'health' drinks and vitamin-enhanced beverages. But does the process of crystallizing magically transform fructose into something healthy? Let's look at the contents. According to the Fructose Information Center (fructose.org), crystalline fructose contains nearly 100 per cent fructose. And just to make it even less appealing, it contains traces of lead, chloride, and arsenic! And keep in mind this information comes from an association that advocates fructose use and consumption.

All of this is very bad news for those who are fructose intolerant and don't even know it. They may suffer from chronic problems such as irritable bowel syndrome without making the connection between their condition and their fructose intake.

• Herbal tea slashes high blood sugar levels by 18% in just 8 weeks

Sheila Danot struggled with type 2 diabetes for nearly 20 years, but despite the cocktail of drugs her doctor put her on she was unable to get her blood sugar levels under control. Then she read about a new tea for diabetes and, despite being extremely sceptical, she bought it to try.

Before she started drinking the tea, her average morning blood sugar level hovered in the high 135-140 range, even though she was taking three pharmaceutical drugs and insulin. But, when she added the tea, her blood sugar dropped dramatically, by around 25 per cent, all the way down to the 100-110 range... sometimes going as low as 97. Even better, her A1c level (more on that in a moment) dropped drastically, from a dangerous 12 down to a much safer 6.7 – a whopping 44 per cent improvement.

"I've been drinking it for a year now and I'll keep drinking it as long as it works, even if my doctor doesn't believe it," she says.

Sheila's doctor may not believe that this healing tea works, but science backs up its effectiveness. Not only are the two key ingredients well studied, the company (called Galilee Tisanes) that makes Glucole put it to the test in a small pilot study involving 10 participants being treated for type 2 diabetes, who were not using insulin. The subjects drank 3 cups of Glucole tea per day with meals without making any other changes. The researchers tracked fasting blood glucose levels and A1c levels every week.

At the start, the average fasting glucose was 180 (healthy fasting sugar levels fall in the 70-130 range). After 8 weeks drinking Glucole, that average dropped a stunning 18.3 per cent down to 147 (still high, but much closer to normal). The tea also brought on a healthy drop in A1c levels, from an average value of 7.2 down to 6.8, back into the safe zone in just 8 weeks. Plus, on average, the participants dropped about 5 pounds over the 8-week study, just from drinking the tea. They also reported fewer food cravings and decreased thirst, two very common symptoms of diabetes.

Controlling A1c means fewer complications

Keeping your blood sugar levels under control is crucial to your long-term health. Too much glucose in your bloodstream can damage your red blood cells (glycosated haemoglobin), and that can lead to very serious complications. So it's really important to keep track of your A1c (also called HbA1c), which tracks those damaged blood cells, and shows a better picture of your sugar levels over the past four months, the typical lifespan of a red blood cell.

Normal A1c levels range from 4-6, and if you have diabetes your doctor probably told you to aim for a level below 7. That's because a score over 7 means you're heading into the danger zone, and the beginnings of possible permanent damage.

The key to sugar control is addressing all the right causes

According to Dr. Zanbar, the man who formulated Glucole: "Many things can cause high blood sugar. The answer depends on the reason for the sugar problem. It can be not enough insulin, or insulin not getting into the cells, or even stress."

To find just the right formula, he tried more than 30 different combinations of herbs before landing on the final six that make up the Glucole formula: Gymnema sylvestre, stevia, olive leaves, sage, lemon verbena and lemon grass. Each of these ingredients works in different ways to counteract each cause of high blood sugar.

Gymnema sylvestre helps regenerate special beta cells in the pancreas, the very cells responsible for producing and secreting insulin. In an animal study, gymnema actually doubled the number of viable beta cells in rats with induced diabetes (*Journal of Ethnopharmacy. 30(3):265-269, 1990*).

In another study, gymnema extract was given to 22 patients with type 2 diabetes along with their prescription medication (*Journal of Ethnopharmacology. 30 (3): 295-305, 1990*). During the 20-month study, researchers saw blood glucose levels and A1c values drop significantly. What's more, five of those diabetic patients were able to completely discontinue using prescription drugs and maintain healthy blood sugar levels with the extract alone. Gymnema can also help reduce carbohydrate cravings and prevent obesity, thanks to its ability to block sweet sensations on your tongue.

Stevia plays an important role in diabetes control

Stevia is much sweeter than sugar and just the tiniest amount acts as a zero-calorie sweetener. Better still, this herb stabilizes blood sugar while it reduces insulin resistance, two key factors in type 2 diabetes.

One small study of 12 patients with type 2 diabetes showed an 18 per cent improvement in glucose management after a test meal (*Metabolism. 53 (1): 73-76, 2004*). The researchers also saw a 40 per cent increase in the insulinogenic index, a scientific ratio that measures insulin sensitivity.

An animal study showed just how stevia impacted blood sugar levels and insulin (*Planta Med. 71 (2): 108-113, 2005*). First, it improved insulin secretion, so there was enough insulin circulating in the blood stream. Second, the insulin worked more effectively, allowing glucose levels to drop. This combination of actions led to lower blood sugar levels within just 90 minutes.

The four remaining herbs increase the effectiveness of Glucole

Olive leaf contains a substance called oleuropein, which helps limit the damage that can be caused by too much sugar circulating in the blood stream.

Sage has a calming effect, which helps combat stress-related increases in blood sugar (*Neuropsychopharmacology. 31 (4): 845-852, 2006*).

Lemon verbena helps ease the signs of physical stress, which can increase blood sugar levels.

Lemon grass helps detoxify the liver, pancreas and kidneys – three organs that can be negatively impacted by diabetes. It also helps promote a sense of calm.

What to take for best results

To help maintain healthy blood sugar levels, drink one or two cups per day with meals. If using just once a day, drink the tea with the heaviest meal. For a more dramatic sugar-controlling effect, drink three cups per day, one after each meal.

• **What's the verdict on coffee drinking and diabetes?**

The advice on whether diabetics should drink coffee or not has been mixed in recent years. Some doctors believe coffee is bad for diabetes sufferers. They claim that the caffeine in coffee stimulates the adrenal glands to produce the hormone adrenalin. This in turn causes the liver to convert some of its store of glycogen into glucose, so raising blood sugar levels. The hike in blood sugar is what gives you the energy boost you expect from a cup of coffee, but, because people with diabetes need to keep their blood sugar stable some argue that they should avoid drinking coffee or have decaffeinated instead.

In the last few years, though, study after study has shown that drinking coffee may actually reduce the risk of type 2 diabetes.

In 2012, a major European study (called EPIC – the European Prospective Investigation into Cancer and Nutrition) reported on the effects of coffee consumption on chronic diseases (*Am J Clin Nutr. 2012 Feb 15. [Epub ahead of print]*). Data from 42,659 participants was collected over a period of nine years, which means that the conclusions drawn from this research are statistically very reliable. People drinking four or more cups of coffee a day had a 23 per cent lower risk of developing type 2 diabetes than those drinking less than one cup a day. If the coffee was decaffeinated, the risk reduction was 30 per cent. Other, smaller studies have suggested levels of risk reduction as high as 50 or 60 per cent.

The EPIC study comes hard on the heels of an animal study at Mount Sinai School of Medicine in New York, in which researchers fed decaffeinated coffee to mice with diet-induced type 2 diabetes for five months (*Nutr Neurosci. 2012; 15(1):37-45*). They found that these mice metabolised glucose and used it for cellular energy in their brains more effectively than mice whose diet was not supplemented with coffee.

Glucose utilisation in the brain is reduced in people with type 2 diabetes, which can result in cognitive problems and may contribute to the development of Alzheimer's disease and other forms of dementia. Further clinical studies in people with diabetes are needed to confirm that the conclusions of this animal study also apply in humans, but this research suggests that, as well as preventing type 2 diabetes, coffee might also help to prevent one of its most distressing complications.

Other animal research has found that coffee consumption prevents the development of high-blood sugar and also improves insulin sensitivity, so reducing the risk of diabetes (*J Agric Food Chem. 2010; 58(9):5597-5603*). Coffee also caused a cascade of other beneficial changes associated with fat metabolism in the liver and the production of inflammatory compounds called adipocytokines, in ways that reduced diabetes risk.

New research shows how coffee might cut the risk of type 2 diabetes

Recent research from China has shed some light on one possible way in which coffee might help to protect against diabetes (*J Agric Food Chem. 2011 Dec 28;59(24):13147-55*). It has to do with a protein called human islet amyloid polypeptide (hIAPP), which is secreted by the pancreas along with the hormone insulin. In people with metabolic syndrome, it seems that this protein, which has a complex three-dimensional structure, becomes distorted or 'misfolded' in a way that leads to the formation of amyloid plaques, comparable to those seen in the brains of Alzheimer's disease patients. These plaques then promote the death of insulin-producing cells in the pancreas, leading to type 2 diabetes.

Compounds in coffee, including caffeine, caffeic acid and chlorogenic acid, were all found to prevent the misfolding of hIAPP and to prevent the accumulation of amyloid plaques. Caffeic acid, which is present in both whole and decaffeinated coffee, had the strongest effect.

So, it appears that coffee really does help to protect against the development of type 2 diabetes and a possible mechanism for this effect has been found. But what if you already have diabetes? Some studies have shown that regular coffee does in fact raise blood sugar levels.

A clinical trial at the University of Guelph, in Canada, gave healthy young men a strong dose of either caffeinated or decaffeinated coffee, followed one hour later by either a high GI or low GI meal (*Am J Clin Nutr. 2008 May; 87 (5): 1254-61*). The subjects then underwent glucose tolerance testing. The results showed that caffeinated coffee significantly impaired blood sugar control and insulin sensitivity, irrespective of the type of meal that was subsequently consumed. Decaffeinated coffee did not have these effects.

The message from these studies seems to be that it is fine to carry on drinking coffee if you are not diabetic. As well as showing a protective effect against type 2 diabetes, the EPIC study also found that it does not increase the risk of heart disease or stroke. However, if you already have type 1 or type 2 diabetes, you may want to switch to decaffeinated instead, which has the same benefits as caffeinated, without the blood sugar disruption.

The following lifestyle changes can help you win the war on diabetes:

- **Exercise can help to stabilise blood sugar levels and improve insulin sensitivity**

We all know that we should do more exercise. In today's high-tech, labour-saving world, exercise is becoming less and less a part of everyday life and increasingly something that we have to consciously find time for. Everybody can benefit from taking regular exercise, but if you are diabetic, it really is a vital element in managing your condition, even if you don't need to lose weight.

That's because regular exercise does more than just keep your weight down, improve your cardiovascular fitness and make you feel good. For those with type 1 diabetes, it lowers blood sugar levels and may help you to reduce the amount of insulin you need. Exercise also tackles the root cause of type 2 diabetes, by reducing insulin resistance, so that glucose is used more effectively.

For people with type 1 or type 2 diabetes, exercising regularly brings other health benefits, too, including the following:

- Improved circulation and reduced cardiovascular risks,

- Lower blood pressure,

- Lower levels of 'bad' cholesterol (LDL) and increased 'good' cholesterol (HDL),

- Increased fat loss and more muscle mass,

- Reduced stress and a more positive outlook,

- Improved brain function.

In just the last few months, several studies have been published that shed more light on the ways in which exercise can prevent or reverse the changes that take place in diabetes.

- **Exercise puts a stop to the inflammatory process behind type 2 diabetes**

Researchers in Greece have been investigating the effects of exercise on adipokines, compounds produced by fat cells that have been described as the 'missing link' between obesity and insulin resistance. The release of adipokines leads to chronic, low level inflammation that is thought to play a central role in the development of insulin resistance and type 2 diabetes (*Diabetes Metab. 2008 Feb; 34(1): 2-11*).

What this clinical study revealed was that you don't have to spend all day in the gym to see beneficial effects. Even moderate exercise for more than two hours a week was associated with significantly lower levels of adipokines and improved blood sugar control, in patients with type 2 diabetes (*Eur J Intern Med. 2012 Mar; 23(2):137-142. Epub 2011 Nov 29*).

Laboratory experiments at the German Diabetes Centre in Dusseldorf have delved further into what goes on in muscle cells exposed to adipokines and how exercise impacts on this process (*Diabetologia. 2012 Jan 27. [Epub ahead of print]*). They found that human muscle cell cultures became insulin resistant when grown in the presence of adipokines. More importantly, this could be overridden by stimulating muscle cells to contract. Contracting muscle cells were far better at taking in glucose in the presence of insulin than were passive cells.

In other words, making your muscles work can reverse insulin resistance, the cause of type 2 diabetes. If there was a pill that could do this as effectively, with no adverse side effects and with a huge list of additional benefits, every doctor in the country would be prescribing it!

Getting more exercise doesn't need to involve a rigorous programme of workouts. A 30 to 40 minute brisk walk, at least three times a week is enough to improve your fitness level and reduce cardiovascular risk. To get the more specific benefits for diabetes, of better blood sugar control and less insulin resistance, try to work some kind of exercise into your routine every day if you can, for instance, by:

- Using stairs instead of a lift or escalator;

- Walking or cycling for short journeys, rather than using the car;

- Getting off the bus or tube a stop early;

- Planning your journey to work to include a walk through a park;

- Using your lunch break to go for a stroll and explore the surrounding area;

- Taking the dog for a walk or taking up an active hobby, such as golf;

- Doing energetic housework, DIY or gardening.

High-intensity interval training hits insulin resistance for six

If you are already exercising and you want an organised training routine that will have maximum impact on your diabetes, the latest research shows that high-intensity interval training can achieve this better than any other form of exercise. Forget spending hours on the treadmill or pounding the pavements. Much more effective, it seems, is a timed workout that alternates moderate exercise with really going for it as hard as you can.

In a small trial at McMaster University, Hamilton, Canada, adults with type 2 diabetes had their blood sugar monitored for 24 hours following high intensity interval training and on a rest day. Following the training session, blood sugar levels remained lower and postprandial hyperglycaemia (the hike in blood sugar levels after a meal) was reduced, compared to rest day readings (*Diabetes Obes Metab. 2012 Jan 23. [Epub ahead of print]*).

The value of this kind of workout lies in the short periods of anaerobic exercise, when your muscles are working so hard that the blood system can't supply them with enough oxygen for normal function. When muscles contract during anaerobic exercise, their ability to take up glucose from the bloodstream is maximised.

A new study at Bedford University has shown that anaerobic exercise (in this case participants exercised while breathing low-oxygen air) is more effective than aerobic exercise in reducing insulin resistance in type 2 diabetic patients (*J Clin Endocrinol Metab. 2012 Jan 25. [Epub ahead of print]*). The improvements seen lasted for 48 hours, following a one-hour workout.

So, if you are not exercising already, you will be amazed at how moving your body more can help you manage your diabetes better. If you are already following an exercise routine, incorporating high-intensity interval training could take the beneficial effects a step further.

Yoga helps reduce inflammation – one of the main culprits behind type 2 diabetes

Inflammation is a key player in many types of chronic disease, including type 2 diabetes. New evidence shows that yoga may be an effective way to control inflammation. Researchers recruited 50 middle aged women who practiced yoga. Half were yoga novices and half were considered advanced with at least two years of consistent yoga practice.

Subjects were put through a series of physical and mental stress tests and blood samples were taken throughout the testing. Analysis showed that an important inflammation marker known as IP-6 that signals risk of type 2 diabetes, heart disease and stroke remained significantly lower among women in the advanced group.

Researchers note that the combination of stretching and exercise in yoga improves flexibility, relaxes the body, and lowers stress – a series of events that helps control inflammation.

• **Sitting for too long increases diabetes risk**

Many of us have jobs that require us to sit for much of the day. In addition, most leisure 'activity' also involves sitting: television, computer games, car travel and even going to the cinema or theatre. Now, scientists at Leicester University have revealed that all that sitting actually increases your risk of diabetes, heart disease and death (*Diabetologia. 2012; 55 (11): 2895-2905*).

We all know that exercise is good for us, but what the latest study has shown is that even if you meet current physical activity guidelines, your health may still be at risk if you remain seated for long periods of time during the day. Not getting enough exercise and sitting for too long are both bad. But they are not the same thing and they affect the body in different ways.

The Leicester University researchers combined the results of 18 studiesinvolving a total of 794,577 participants. Their meta-analysis showed that, compared with those who sat the least, people whose sedentary time was longest had a 112 per cent increased risk of diabetes and a 147 per cent increased risk of a cardiovascular event. They also had a 90 per cent greater chance of dying from a heart attack or stroke. The strength of these associations was most consistent for diabetes – that is to say, the more time you spend sitting, the more likely you are to develop type 2 diabetes, even if you work out at the gym three times a week.

As startling as these findings are, the idea is not new. Professor Frank Booth, at the University of Missouri, coined the term 'sedentary death syndrome' in 2004, to describe the public health burden of chronic disease arising from a society where sitting for most of the day is the norm (*Can J Appl Physiol. 2004; 29 (4): 447-460*). Professor Booth considers physical inactivity to be a disease in itself, resulting in pathological changes in the body.

In particular, prolonged sitting reduces the uptake of glucose by muscle cells, leading to higher blood sugar levels. In addition, sitting for long periods of time appears to suppress the production of new nerve cells in the specific parts of the brain that are responsible for memory, motor skill learning and the urge to meet survival needs.

How many breaks you take is more important than the total time spent sitting

The good thing is that just by taking frequent breaks from sitting down you can start to reverse these increased risks. Even if you have to spend a long time sitting down during the day in total, breaking it up with short periods of standing or moving around can make a big difference (*Exerc Sport Sci Rev. 2010; 38 (3): 105-113*). Standing uses postural muscles that are not engaged during sitting, so just standing and chatting with somebody during your coffee break can help.

Here are some other tips for avoiding prolonged, inactive sitting and the health risks it entails:

- Sit up straight – this works core muscles in your back and abdomen; if your workplace allows, sit on an exercise ball instead of a chair to activate the muscles that keep you balanced.

- Do isotonics – while sitting, press alternate feet down against the floor to contract thigh muscles; work your gluteals by clenching your buttocks, too.

- If you use an electronic organiser, set reminders at 45 minute intervals throughout the day, so that you don't forget to stand up and move around frequently.

- Put your laptop on the filing cabinet and work standing up for a while.

- Try to hold conversations standing up. This is also a good way to keep meetings short!

- When watching television, get into the habit of getting up and doing something else during the ads and the breaks between programmes.

- For short journeys, walk or cycle instead of taking the car.

- Choose leisure activities that really are active – for instance, take your children or grandchildren to the ice rink instead of to the cinema; or have a walk in the park with your friends instead of sitting in the coffee shop.

Reducing the amount of time you spend sitting will cut your risk of developing type 2 diabetes and will also reduce your risk of cardiovascular disease. If you already have diabetes, it will help by reducing insulin resistance and keeping blood sugar more stable.

• How getting a good night's sleep can help prevent type 2 diabetes

When it comes to lifestyle changes for managing diabetes, most of us are aware of the importance of eating sensibly and getting enough exercise. But there is another lifestyle factor that can have a dramatic effect on diabetes: sleep.

Each of us has a body clock, which tells us when we need to sleep and when to get up. It also controls the timing of metabolic processes in the body throughout the day and night. In the morning, daylight triggers the production of the hormones cortisol and serotonin, to wake us up and raise both blood pressure and body temperature. As darkness falls, the pineal gland in the brain starts to secrete the 'sleep hormone' melatonin and blood pressure falls as the body prepares for a night's rest.

Anybody who has experienced jet lag knows how strong an effect our body clock has on the way we function and how bad we feel when it is out of kilter. But feeling fatigued, disorientated and unable to concentrate are just the outward signs of disruption to our daily rhythm; the internal effects are more serious and may lead to obesity, insulin resistance, high blood pressure and type 2 diabetes (*Cardiovasc Diabetol 2011; 10: 24*).

Scientists have known for a long time that people who work night shifts are more likely than day workers to gain weight and to develop metabolic syndrome and diabetes. In the last couple of years, we have started to find out why.

Glucocorticoid hormones are produced in the adrenal glands and play an important role in the regulation of blood sugar levels. The most important one is cortisol. Recent research has discovered that daily fluctuations in glucocorticoid levels directly synchronise the biological clock as an integral part of our mechanism for regulating blood sugar (*Proc Natl Acad Sci USA 2009; 106 (41): 17582-17587*). In other words, if we don't produce cortisol at the right times of day and in the right amounts, our blood sugar control suffers.

The same genetic factors influence your body clock and your diabetes risk

The results of a new genetic study published in January 2012 have added to knowledge from earlier research on the roles that mutations to specific genes play in this relationship between body clocks and diabetes. The production of melatonin, a hormone that is a key player in setting the timing of our body clocks, is controlled by a series of genes. The international research, led by a team at Imperial College, London, has found that abnormal variations in these genes increase the risk of developing type 2 diabetes, in some cases by 600 per cent (*Nat Genet. 2012 Jan 29. [Epub ahead of print]; Nat Genet. 2009 Jan;41 (1): 89-94*).

Of course, susceptibility to type 2 diabetes has long been suspected of having a genetic factor, since there is a tendency for it to run in families. And there is not much you can do to change your genes. You can, however, make a difference to your body's production of the hormones involved in regulating your body clock, so that your blood sugar control improves as a consequence.

The main thing you can do to ensure a good production of melatonin at night is to keep to a regular bedtime and waking time. It's also important to sleep in a dark room, so get thick curtains if outside light sources are illuminating your bedroom. When getting ready for bed, use a dim bedside light, just enough to see by, and don't watch television or use a computer in bed. If you need to get up in the night don't switch on the light unless it's essential. During the daytime, it also helps to get as much natural daylight as possible.

These simple steps can help to ensure that your body produces enough melatonin to effectively regulate both your body clock and your blood sugar. Avoiding overproduction of the 'wake-up' hormone cortisol before bedtime is equally important, so avoid stressful situations and violent television programmes or video games late in the evening.

Chapter 4

These all-natural breakthroughs can help reduce your blood sugar levels

The following supplements and herbal remedies have all been proven to be effective in the fight against diabetes and metabolic syndrome. Some have additional benefits, such as lowering high blood pressure and triglyceride (blood fat) levels, which can help ward off diabetic complications like heart disease. In fact, some of these remedies are so effective that they can banish the need for medication altogether in some cases.

However, it is extremely important that you do not stop taking any prescribed medication without consulting your doctor first. It's also vital that you consult your doctor if you're currently on any medication prior to taking these remedies, in order to prevent any possible contraindications. Taking them in combination with other blood sugar lowering therapies may lower your blood sugar levels too far and your doctor may need to reduce your injected insulin or diabetes medications. So, it's crucial to monitor your progress closely with the help of a medical professional.

Even if you are not taking any medication it is still vital that you keep your doctor fully informed of any natural remedies you decide to take, as your blood sugar levels need to be closely monitored.

In addition, it is important to realise that there is no telling which treatment, or combination of treatments, will work best for you. While one supplement can produce noticeable improvements in one individual, it may have little or no effect on another person.

Likewise, natural remedies can take longer to work than conventional drugs in some cases. For this reason, you should allow enough time for a supplement to work properly. It may be the case that you have to try a few different treatments before you find one that works for you.

It is also important that any nutritional supplement or herbal remedy be taken in conjunction with regular exercise and a healthy low GL diet that is low in sugar and refined carbohydrates (like white bread and pasta) which can rapidly cause your blood sugar levels to soar.

- ## Why a simple fruit extract could be set to replace conventional drugs for treating diabetes

The bitter melon plant (*Momordica charantia*) can be found growing in tropical locations such as East Africa, Asia, The Caribbean and South America – where its fruit is used both as a medicine and a food, and as the name suggests, it tastes bitter.

Mounting research into bitter melon's unique therapeutic properties is an example of the advantages natural therapies can have over conventional drugs. In India, doctors are so confident about the anti-diabetic effect of bitter melon that it is often dispensed in hospitals to people suffering from diabetes in place of medication. Similarly in Myanmar (Burma), the plant is prescribed by traditional physicians to diabetic patients, and in China it is used for the same purpose.

It is the extract from the unripe fruit that provides the plant with its therapeutic properties. At least 32 active constituents have been identified in bitter melon so far, including 5-hydroxytryptamine, beta-sitosterol-d-glucoside, citrulline, cryptoxanthin, GABA, lutein, lycopene and zeaxanthin. Nutritional analysis reveals that bitter melon is also rich in potassium, calcium, iron and beta-carotene. It also contains vitamins B1, B2, B3 and C.

Not only is bitter melon proving highly effective for lowering blood sugar levels, but animal studies have found that it can help reduce body fat too. Chinese researchers working at the Department of Zoology, University of Hong Kong, have found that bitter melon improves fat metabolism and can significantly reduce abdominal fat in diabetic animals that are also obese (*J Nutr 2003, 133 (4): 1088-1093*).

Again, this has important implications for diabetic patients who have a tendency to accumulate fat, particularly around the abdominal area, as a result of an inability to utilise fat efficiently.

Bitter melon found to be even more effective than a conventional drug in lowering blood sugar

The Department of Health in the Philippines has recommended bitter melon as one of the best herbal medicines for diabetic management. Plus, multiple clinical studies have clearly established the role of bitter melon in people with diabetes (*Phytomed 1996; 2: 349-62*).

A study conducted to assess the effectiveness of bitter melon and exercise for type 2 diabetes, revealed how taking both these measures can significantly lower blood sugar levels (*Miura T, Itoh Y et al. Biol Pharm Bull 2004, 27 (2): 248-250*). Not only that but it has also been found to be just as effective as the prescription only drug glibenclamide at reducing blood sugar levels (*J Ethnopharmacol 2003, 88 (1): 107-111*).

A clinical trial, in which researchers compared the effects in diabetes patients of a bitter melon extract and the now-banned drug Avandia (rosiglitazone), showed that bitter melon could be more effective in the management of diabetes and its related complications (*Phytomedicine. 2009; 16 (5): 401-405*). Avandia was subsequently banned in the EU as it was linked with an increased risk of heart attacks.

Scientists have identified three groups of constituents in bitter melon that are thought to be responsible for its 'blood sugar lowering' action. One of these, a compound called charantin, which is composed of mixed steroids, was found to be more effective than the oral hypoglycaemic drug tolbutamide in reducing blood sugar.

Another, an insulin-like polypeptide called polypeptide-P, appears to lower blood sugar in type 1 diabetics, while alkaloids present in the fruit have also been noted to have a blood sugar lowering effect. As yet, researchers are unclear as to which of these compounds is most effective or if it is the synergistic effect of all three. Further research is required to understand how these compounds actually work.

Compounds known as oleanolic acid glycosides have been found to improve glucose tolerance in type 2 diabetic patients by preventing the absorption of sugar from the intestines. Bitter melon has also been reported to increase the number of beta cells (cells that secrete insulin) in the pancreas, thereby improving the body's capability to produce insulin, which promotes the uptake of sugar from the blood by cells and tissues. Due to bitter melon's effect on beta cells, it is one of the few agents with the potential to rejuvenate a flagging pancreas.

In one study, glucose tolerance was improved in 73 per cent of type 2 diabetics given 2oz of bitter melon juice (*J Ethnopharmacol 1986; 17: 277-282*). In another study, 15 grams of the aqueous extract of bitter melon produced a 54 per cent decrease in post-prandial (occurring after eating) blood sugar in six patients (*Phytother Res 1993; 7: 285-289*).

Bitter melon also helps defend against diabetes-related complications

Dozens of studies have shown that bitter melon is effective, both in terms of reducing blood sugar levels and preventing diabetes-related complications (*Fitotherapia 2003, 74 (1-2): 7-13*). For example, an animal study performed at the All India Institute of Medical Sciences revealed that the fruit extract was able to reduce the risk of cataracts – a well-known diabetic complication – by almost 100 per cent, following just four months of treatment (*Phytother Res 2002 16 (8): 774-777*).

Following a large review study, which assessed the effectiveness of various plant remedies for treating diabetes, scientists from the Division for Research and Education in Complementary and Integrative Medical Therapies at Harvard Medical School, claimed that bitter melon was one of the best herbal remedies for fighting the condition.

The scientists reviewed all of the available medical literature on plants and supplements for diabetes – in total these studies involved 4,565 diabetic patients. The final conclusion was that bitter melon, alongside other plants like Gymnema sylvestre, was extremely beneficial in terms of lowering blood sugar levels and preventing diabetes-related complications (*Diabetes Care 2003, 26 (4): 1277-1294*).

Get all the benefits of bitter melon without its bitter taste

Bitter melon has been a folk remedy for high blood sugar for many years. But this medicinal vegetable didn't come by its name by accident, and most people are put off by the taste – no matter what the benefits. But one supplier from the Philippines has perfected a method of capturing the beneficial phytochemicals from bitter melon while removing the notorious bitter taste in their bitter melon products, which are called Charantia. After hearing promising things about Charantia, Dr. Guia Abad, the president of the Association of Municipal Health Officers of the Philippines (AMHOP), decided to try it for her own blood sugar problems.

Years ago, before Charantia products were available, Dr. Abad used to buy actual bitter melons and prepare them for herself and her husband to eat, to help them both control their blood sugar levels. At that time, folk wisdom taught, "the more bitter, the better," suggesting that the worst-tasting bitter melon would impart the most benefits. So Dr. Abad was sceptical when she first heard of this pleasant tasting Charantia tea.

But she decided to try it anyway, since she has a strong family history of diabetes. After just a short time, she had to reduce the amount of Charantia she was drinking, because her blood sugar level was sinking too low. After her positive experiences, she began recommending Charantia to her patients and colleagues. "It has been very effective," Dr. Abad says. "It has helped [a lot of my patients] control their expenses, because it reduces their need for expensive drugs." Most of her patients have been able to cut back on their prescription diabetes medications, and some have come off of them entirely.

How to take bitter melon for maximum results

Bitter melon is available from some Asian grocery stores, however due to its bitter taste, you may prefer to take it in an alternative form. There are three varieties of Charantia products available in the UK, all based on the basic ingredient of the dried fruits and seeds of bitter melon: 'Charantia Loose T-Bits' features sliced dried fruit and seeds, which can be steeped in hot water to make a drink; Charantia Tea Bags; and 500mg Charantia Capsules. No matter what way you prefer to take Charantia, it's important to follow the specific dosage amounts given on the individual product's label or as otherwise directed by your practitioner. All of the Charantia products should be taken after a meal, not on an empty stomach.

WARNING: Individuals with hypoglycaemia (low blood sugar) should not take bitter melon (*Momordica charantia*) as it is likely to aggravate the problem. It is also important to note that because bitter melon alters blood sugar status so effectively, those with diabetes should take it only under the supervision of their GP. Bitter melon is also contraindicated during pregnancy. The intake of excessive amounts of bitter melon juice may cause diarrhoea.

• **Goat's rue has similar clinical benefits to conventional diabetes drugs but without their unpleasant side effects**

A wealth of research now exists to support the remarkable anti-diabetic properties of a plant called goat's rue. It has also been found to promote weight-loss, prevent the formation of dangerous blood clots (*J Ethnopharmacol 2000, 69 (3): 235-240*), and act as a powerful anti-bacterial agent (*J Ethnopharmacol 2001, 77 (1): 111-112*).

Goat's rue contains the chemical galegin, which is key to its extraordinary anti-diabetic effects. Galegin is chemically very similar to another agent called guanidine, the standard compound from which many conventional diabetic drugs are manufactured, such as metformin (*Phytother Res 1999, 13 (2): 91-94*).

However, because goat's rue is a plant, it has fewer side effects than synthetic drugs such as metformin, which can cause loss of appetite, nausea, vomiting, stomach pains and diarrhoea.

Dr. Ward Dean, a member of the Board of Directors of the American Academy of Anti-Aging Medicine, is responsible for much of the original research on goat's rue and diabetes. Following extensive studies, he believes that goat's rue has the same clinical benefits as metformin (*Vitamin Research News 2001, 15 (3): 4-5*).

Goat's rue reduces the threat of diabetes-related complications developing

Diabetes is characterised by too much glucose in the blood. Over time, high levels of blood glucose can cause irreparable damage to body tissue, particularly your eyes, peripheral nerves, kidneys and veins, as well as suppressing your immune system.

Scientists have discovered that goat's rue initiates a reduction in blood glucose levels (without triggering the symptoms of hypoglycaemia); and reduces the risk of cataracts and retinopathy (degeneration of your retina), and kidney damage which is common among diabetics. It also slows down the advance of atherosclerosis (*Vitamin Research News 2001, 15 (3): 4-5; Experimental Eye Rearch 1996, 62; 505-510*).

Exactly how goat's rue works is still unknown, but some scientists believe it is able to influence diabetes through its 'receptor sensitising' activities. The production of major hormones, such as insulin, is dependent upon the communication between cells and other stimulatory hormones and chemicals. The point of contact between the hormone or chemical and the cell is called the membrane receptor.

As you age, the responsiveness of these receptors declines. This means that your cells are not stimulated enough and become inactive, which results in inadequate amounts of insulin (and other hormones) being produced.

Receptor sensitisers, such as goat's rue, are nutrients and chemicals that have the ability to rejuvenate your membrane receptors, making your cells more responsive to hormonal and chemical stimulation. Goat's rue helps restore insulin sensitivity in your cells, and boosts their ability to take up glucose from your blood and use it more efficiently (*Vitamin Research News 2001, 15 (10); 1-16*).

In addition, animal studies carried out by scientists, at the Department of Pharmaceutical Sciences at Strathclyde University in Glasgow, found that goat's rue can cause a significant reduction in body weight (*J Pharm Pharmacol 1999, 51 (11): 1313-1319*). More astonishing still was that this weight loss was maintained even after treatment with goat's rue had stopped and a normal diet resumed.

What to take for best results

The recommended dosage of goat's rue is 200mg a day, or as otherwise directed on the product's label. As mentioned previously, please consult your doctor before trying goat's rue, especially if you are already taking medication.

• Why antioxidants are so vital for diabetes sufferers

One of the biggest advances in medical science in recent years has been the growing appreciation that ageing, chronic inflammation, obesity and medical conditions such as diabetes and heart disease all share a common cause. This is the phenomenon known as oxidative stress.

Normal biological functions naturally produce highly reactive molecules called free radicals, also called 'reactive oxygen species'. These molecules have toxic or damaging effects in the body, which are counteracted by antioxidants that the body produces or that are present in foods. There is a constant war going on between the free radical 'bad guys' and the antioxidant 'good guys'. When there is insufficient antioxidant capacity to balance out the effects of the free radicals, the result is oxidative stress. Many scientists now believe that almost all of the disease processes in the body involve oxidative stress as a 'final common pathway' (*Rev Diabet Stud. 2010; 7 (1): 15-25*).

The three ways oxidative stress makes diabetes worse

As mentioned on page 101, oxidative stress is involved in three main ways when it comes to diabetes: It damages the insulin-producing beta-cells in the pancreas; contributes to insulin resistance; and causes changes to blood vessels that result in diabetic complications (heart disease, kidney damage and eye problems). It is also involved in obesity and high blood pressure, two conditions that frequently accompany diabetes (*Clin Chem Lab Med. 2011; 49 (11): 1773-1782*).

High levels of blood sugar and blood fats cause oxidative stress in the pancreatic beta-cells, which produce insulin. The beta-cells are especially vulnerable to this kind of damage, which results in lowered output of insulin and increased cell death (*Pflugers Arch. 2010; 460(4):703-718*). This means that the pancreas cannot always produce sufficient insulin to deal with the level of sugar in the blood, leading to chronic high sugar levels which are in turn a cause of further oxidative stress. In this way a 'vicious cycle' of damage to the pancreas is set up.

Oxidative stress also interferes with the way in which insulin acts in the body. Like other hormones, insulin provides chemical signals to cells to instruct them to act in particular ways. In the case of insulin, the instruction is to make changes to the cell membrane in order to allow glucose or fat to pass through into the cell. Oxidative stress changes the structure of specific proteins that are key to the way this insulin signalling system works (*Free Radic Biol Med. 2011; 50 (5): 567-575*). The outcome is that the cells no longer respond to insulin, a condition called insulin resistance and the underlying cause of type 2 diabetes.

The third way in which oxidative stress is relevant to diabetes is in causing many of the complications associated with it. Oxidative stress is a direct cause of vascular dysfunction, an abnormal condition of the blood vessels that leads in turn to plaque formation in the arteries and consequent risk of cardiovascular disease (*Postgrad Med J. 2003; 79:195-200*). It also damages blood vessels in the kidneys and eyes, causing diabetic nephropathy (kidney disease) and retinopathy (loss of vision).

To avoid oxidative stress and its damaging and degenerative effects, the balance between free radicals and antioxidants has to be loaded in favour of the 'good guys.' This means eating foods and taking supplements that either provide antioxidants directly or stimulate the body to make its own. Top of the list is a compound called glutathione, which the body produces as its primary antioxidant. However, people with diabetes have low levels of glutathione because they are unable to manufacture enough of it (*Int J Mol Med. 2012; 29 (5): 899-905*).

Take these antioxidant supplements

The raw materials for producing glutathione are the amino-acids cysteine, glutamic acid and glycine. Until recently, the best way to boost glutathione levels was to take a supplement of a form of cysteine called N-acetyl cysteine, or NAC. Glutathione could not be used directly as a supplement because it is very poorly absorbed by the digestive system and is rapidly broken down before it reaches the bloodstream. But now a new, stable form of glutathione has been developed, called S-acetyl-L-glutathione, and it is available as a supplement in the UK.

Vitamin C is another essential antioxidant that has been shown to both reduce the risk of developing diabetes and to reduce blood sugar and cholesterol levels in people with the condition. In a recent clinical trial, supplementing with 1,000mg of vitamin C a day resulted in significantly lower fasting blood sugar and glycosylated haemoglobin (a measure of long-term blood sugar control) readings in people with diabetes who were also taking the medication metformin (*Adv Pharmacol Sci. 2011; 2011: 195271*).

For vitamin C to work properly and to be recycled back into an active form after performing its antioxidant function, it needs another antioxidant, called alpha lipoic acid. This brilliant substance also protects your arteries, kidneys, nerves and eyes from the damage caused by too much sugar in the bloodstream. Clinical trials have shown clear benefits of taking additional alpha lipoic acid for people with type 1 and type 2 diabetes, particularly in treating diabetic neuropathy (nerve damage) (*Front Pharmacol. 2011; 2: 69*).

- **Discover how vitamin D can benefit diabetes sufferers**

Several research studies have shown that low levels of vitamin D are linked to the development of insulin resistance and diabetes. In a meta-analysis of 19 separate studies, US scientists at Tufts Medical Centre in Boston, concluded that people with the highest vitamin D status had a 43 per cent lower risk of developing type 2 diabetes, compared to those with the lowest levels of the vitamin (*Eur J Clin Nutr. 2011 Sep; 65(9): 1005-1015*).

This lends support to the finding of a 2008 review, that adequate intake of vitamin D may prevent or delay the onset of diabetes, as well as reducing complications for those who have already been diagnosed (*Diabetes Educ. 2008 Nov-Dec; 34 (6): 939-40, 942, 944 passim*).

A new study has found that obese children with lower vitamin D levels have higher degrees of insulin resistance, further suggesting that vitamin D deficiency may play a role in the development of type 2 diabetes (*J Clin Endocrinol Metab. 2011 Nov 9. [Epub ahead of print]*). So, what's going on?

Well, the first thing to understand about vitamin D is that it isn't really a vitamin at all; that is to say it is not an essential factor in the diet, like vitamin C. We make vitamin D in our skin in the presence of sunlight and chemically it is a secosteroid, very similar to the body's steroid hormones, such as cortisol. Like those hormones, vitamin D locks onto receptors on the surfaces of many types of cells and influences their activity.

A Finnish study has found a clear link between vitamin D intake during the first year of life and the subsequent development of type 1 diabetes (*Lancet. 2001 Nov 3; 358 (9292): 1500-3*). Babies given 2,000 IU of vitamin D daily were at significantly lower risk of developing the disease.

Since then, US researchers at the University of California, San Diego School of Medicine, have established a correlation between people's blood levels of vitamin D and the subsequent incidence of type 1 diabetes (*Diabetologia. 2012; 55 (12): 3224-3227*). So, for the first time, getting a blood test for vitamin D could give an accurate indication of the risk of this condition and how much your blood level might need to be raised to prevent it.

In type 1 diabetes, the immune system destroys the body's own pancreatic beta-cells, which produce insulin. Recent research suggests that vitamin D is instrumental in the production of regulatory T-cells, which instruct the immune system not to attack the body (*Diabetes Metab Res Rev. 2011 Nov 27(8): 942-5*).

The way that vitamin D works to prevent type 2 diabetes is different. In this case, it both promotes insulin production and maintains the sensitivity of cells to insulin (*Diabetes Obes Metab. 2008 Mar; 10 (3): 185-97*). Vitamin D has a direct action on pancreatic beta-cell function and also regulates blood calcium levels, which in turn influence the rate at which insulin is produced and secreted. Deficiency of vitamin D is a contributory factor in insulin resistance and glucose intolerance. In one clinical trial, vitamin D supplementation reduced susceptibility to type 2 diabetes by slowing the loss of insulin sensitivity in people showing early signs of the disease (*Diabetes Care 2007; 30 (4): 980-986*).

Vitamin D is not only important for helping to control blood sugar and insulin levels. It can also help to bring down high blood pressure and triglyceride levels and reduce the build-up of arterial plaque, all of which are risk factors for heart disease and are common complications of diabetes.

Scientists have discovered how, without sufficient vitamin D, immune cells called macrophages bind to blood vessels near the heart and then trap cholesterol to block those blood vessels (*J Biol Chem. 2012; 287 (46): 38482-38494*).

Crucially, the researchers found that having high blood pressure, being overweight, or having high cholesterol or blood sugar levels made little difference to this process. Only vitamin D levels determined whether those cells stuck to the blood vessel walls or not. This means that doing all the right things to make sure your other risk factors are reduced as far as possible may not help much if your vitamin D level is low.

Vitamin D also appears to be involved in the body's weight control and fat metabolism mechanisms. A study has shown that low levels of vitamin D correlate with a higher body mass index and more body fat.

What to take for best results

Taking a vitamin D supplement is a good idea for everybody in the UK, where we just don't get enough strong sunshine for our bodies to make all the vitamin D we need (and many of us avoid the sun anyway because we're worried about skin cancer). For people with diabetes, vitamin D supplementation should be considered an essential part of managing the condition and avoiding its dangerous complications.

Currently, there is no official guidance on how much vitamin D people with diabetes should take. The Department of Health recommends that people who are not exposed to sunlight and people over 65 should take 10 micrograms (equivalent to 400IU) per day. This is not enough to provide for the body's needs without adequate sun exposure, which few of us are able to get.

Make sure you supplement with vitamin D3, also known as cholecalciferol or calcitriol. Researchers involved in the study on vitamin D's role in preventing type 1 diabetes consider that most people would need to take 4,000IU a day of vitamin D3 in order to achieve high enough blood levels to reduce their risk of the disease. Given the wide range of functions that vitamin D has in the body that now seems to be a realistic dose for general good health.

In addition, on those days when the sun does shine, try to get 20 minutes of skin exposure without sunscreen. Eating oily fish is the best way to get extra vitamin D in your diet and it will also provide essential omega-3 fatty acids that have multiple health benefits, including lowering the risk of heart disease.

• How calcium, magnesium and chromium can benefit diabetics

Three key mineral nutrients – calcium, magnesium and chromium – can help keep your blood sugar levels stable:

Calcium

Calcium is best known for keeping bones strong, but it actually has many other roles in the body. A study published in January 2012, involving more than 8,000 people, confirmed earlier findings that those people with the most calcium in their diets have the lowest risk of developing metabolic syndrome (*Am J Clin Nutr 2012; 95 (1): 231-40*).

In an earlier, placebo-controlled trial involving 20 non-diabetic patients with high blood pressure, taking a supplement of 1,500mg of calcium per day for eight weeks was found to improve insulin sensitivity (*Hypertension 1997; 29: 531–536*). A narrow range of calcium ion (Ca^{2+}) concentration within the cell is critical for processes that involve the hormone insulin.

The best food sources of calcium are dairy products, tinned fish (with bones), tofu, nuts, seeds, dried beans and leafy greens. It makes sense to eat these foods on a regular basis, but if you are unable to get your calcium this way, then you may want to opt for a supplement of 1,000mg a day, preferably as calcium citrate, which is more easily absorbed than calcium carbonate.

Magnesium

Magnesium also appears to play a significant role in insulin sensitivity. A review published in *Diabetes Care* last year concluded that higher magnesium intake reduces the incidence of type 2 diabetes (*Diabetes Care*

2011; 34: 2116-2122). The results suggested that this association is much stronger in overweight individuals, who are generally at higher risk of developing the condition.

In a new clinical study published earlier this year, people with type 2 diabetes were found to have significantly lower levels of magnesium than non-diabetic subjects (*PLoS One 2012; 7 (1): e30599*). Forty eight per cent of those with type 2 diabetes had serum magnesium levels below normal, compared to people without diabetes.

This is more likely to reflect the fact that diabetes disrupts magnesium metabolism, causing more to be expelled in the urine, than any difference in magnesium intake. However, it means that if you have type 2 diabetes, you need to get extra magnesium from your diet or take supplements, to make up for the loss.

Nuts, bran, oatmeal, dried beans, spinach, peanut butter, bananas and raisins are all good sources of magnesium. If your diet is low in these foods, you could take a supplement of 300mg to 500mg a day, as magnesium citrate.

Chromium

Chromium is a trace element that is essential for normal carbohydrate and fat metabolism. In fact, insulin simply cannot work properly without it. Studies show that people with type 2 diabetes have lower blood levels of chromium than those without the disease (*Diabetes Educ. 2004; Suppl: 2-14*).

Most of the clinical trials conducted have demonstrated that chromium supplements enhance the metabolic action of insulin. However, some studies have failed to find a beneficial effect and the official line is still that "more research is needed" (despite chromium's blood sugar lowering effects being known since the 1950s!).

The reason for these inconsistent results may be that a clinical response to chromium, in terms of a drop in blood sugar and improved insulin sensitivity, is seen more strongly in patients whose diabetes is less well controlled (*Curr Diab Rep 2010; 10 (2): 145-151*).

Good food sources of chromium are brewer's yeast, lean meat, liver, kidney, cheese, chicken, whole grain products, wheat germ, oatmeal, lentils and mushrooms. However, if you have type 1 or type 2 diabetes, or need to control your blood sugar levels better, it is probably worth taking a supplement of 200mcg a day, in the form of chromium picolinate.

If you take chromium, magnesium or calcium supplements, you may find that you need to reduce injected insulin or diabetes medications. Always talk to your doctor before starting or altering any supplement regime.

• Alpha lipoic acid controls diabetes and its complications

As mentioned previously, oxidative stress plays a big role in damaging the insulin-producing beta-cells in the pancreas and contributing to insulin resistance and diabetic complications. Oxidative stress occurs when the body's antioxidant capacity is insufficient to balance out the damaging effects of free radicals.

Alpha lipoic acid (ALA) is an important antioxidant that can prevent and combat oxidative stress. A recent flurry of research findings has shown that it could in fact be a serious alternative to conventional drugs for the management of diabetes.

Alpha lipoic acid (ALA) helps vitamin C to do its job efficiently by recycling it back into an active form once it has neutralised harmful free radicals. However, studies are showing that it does a great deal more than this. It is also capable of protecting vulnerable tissues in the arteries, nerves, eyes and kidneys from being damaged by oxidation and glycation.

Glycation is a process in which high blood sugar levels cause glucose molecules to attach themselves to proteins, so disrupting their functions in the body. The result is compounds called advanced glycation end products, or AGEs, which impair nerve function, contribute to plaque build-up in the arteries, clog neural pathways in the brain and destroy capillaries in the kidneys and the eyes. Glycation and oxidation also damage the insulin receptors on muscle cells, so making them insulin resistant. ALA protects the body from AGEs and oxidation damage, which together lie behind many of the problems associated with diabetes.

A new clinical trial, carried out in Thailand, has shown just how effective ALA is for improving blood sugar control in diabetes. Patients with diagnosed type 2 diabetes were given varying doses of ALA (300, 600, 900, and 1,200mg/day) or placebo for 6 months and were tested for blood sugar levels and oxidative biomarkers throughout the study (*Asia Pac J Clin Nutr. 2012; 21 (1): 12-21*). The results showed that fasting blood glucose and HbA1c (glycosylated haemoglobin, an indication of both long-term blood sugar levels and glycation damage) decreased in a dose-dependent manner in the group taking ALA. Oxidative stress (free radical damage) increased in the placebo group, but not with ALA treatment.

New studies show ALA protects eyes, kidneys, nerves and heart

These results show that ALA could offer a safe and natural alternative to diabetes drugs, for the control of blood sugar. But the benefits of ALA don't stop there. In just the last few months, study after study has been published demonstrating that this natural nutrient could prevent or improve diabetes and its complications.

The mechanism by which it protects insulin-producing beta cells in the pancreas has been confirmed and clarified. ALA has been shown to protect Schwann cells in the peripheral nervous system, potentially preventing diabetic neuropathy, a condition for which no treatment currently exists. It has also been found to prevent the worsening of retinopathy (eye damage) in diabetes, caused by high doses of insulin, and to delay the deterioration of kidney function in diabetic rats.

Other new research focuses on ALA's ability to prevent damage to the heart and arteries, which is one of the biggest worries for diabetes patients. It has been recommended as a treatment for diabetic cardiomyopathy, in which the heart muscle cells become damaged. It has also been shown to reduce inflammation of the endothelial cells lining the arteries and to reduce or prevent the process of atherosclerosis (hardening of the arteries).

If all this isn't enough to persuade you of ALA's benefits, it could also help you to lose weight. In a new animal study, giving doses of ALA to diabetic mice fed on a high-fat diet dramatically reduced their body weight and visceral fat content. The amount of visceral fat you have (the kind that collects around your body organs) is a reliable indicator of insulin sensitivity, impaired glucose tolerance, high blood pressure and high cholesterol and blood fat levels.

Talk to your doctor about taking an ALA supplement, to establish a dosage that is right for you and that could allow you to reduce other medication you are taking. As a guide, some studies have found significant benefits from a dosage of 600mg a day.

- **Blood sugar plummets by 107 points in just 90 days with this ground-breaking diabetes breakthrough**

If the latest natural diabetes breakthrough, Syntra5, did even half of what it claims, it would still be better than most of the diabetes drugs currently on the market. This ground-breaking formula is twice as effective as some top-selling diabetes drugs at lowering blood glucose in every measure. Plus, it works much, much faster – we're talking days, not months.

One small company goes all in to gamble on a clinical trial

Inspired by all the success stories pouring in from grateful customers who'd used Syntra5, Ken Hampshire, owner of the US-based company Syntratech, wanted to know exactly what his formula could do, so he commissioned a small study involving 17 participants to see how it fared. The results were so positive that Ken decided to take a major gamble and pay for a clinical trial... putting his company on the line. If Syntra5 wasn't proven effective, they would be ruined.

The results were nothing short of ground-breaking:

- Fasting blood sugar plummeted an unheard of average 107 points in just 90 days

- Two-hour glucose levels decreased 54.55%

- HbA1c dropped from an average of 7.7% to 4.7%, a remarkable 3 point drop

- LDL cholesterol decreased by more than 34%

- Total cholesterol dropped over 29%

- Triglycerides fell by 20%

- Systolic blood pressure decreased by 28.4%, along with a 4.9% drop in diastolic blood pressure

- Average weight loss was 9.3 pounds – with NO changes in eating or exercise

And those were the results after only 90 days, in patients with chronic uncontrolled blood glucose and fasting blood glucose counts between 160 mg/dL and 225 mg/dL (a definite danger zone) (*Human Clinical Trial Evaluating the Safety and Efficacy of Diatroxal® A Randomized, Double-Blind Placebo Controlled Study, research and report by: Melonie Montgomery, MSHN, Director of Research, Fenestra Research Labs* (*unpublished study, commissioned by Syntratech™ Corporation*)).

During the clinical trial, they also ran a glucose challenge test, loading the subjects with 75 grams of glucose (that's about 6 tablespoons) to see the response. Of course, when you take in that much sugar, your blood glucose spikes up, and it may take a long time to level out (the standard measure of how well the body handles sugar after eating is a two-hour test). Yet, almost everyone in the Syntra5 group had normalized blood sugar within 30 minutes of the glucose load!

Syntra5 is getting results that Big Pharma can only dream about

If you've got diabetes, you aim for normal zone numbers: Fasting blood glucose under 100 mg/dL; 2-hour glucose level under 140 mg/dL; HbA1c level under 7%.

HbA1c is one of the most important numbers in diabetes management because it measures long-term glucose control. Leading diabetes drugs can't really lower HbA1c by very much (one of the biggest decreases is 1.4 with metformin), or get that number under the 7% benchmark. However, in the **clinical trial, 100% of patients taking Syntra5 saw their HbA1c drop to 5%**. In just 90 days... and that was down from an average 7.7% at the start of the trial.

Then there's the fasting glucose level. Top-selling diabetes drugs only drop blood glucose levels by around 50 points. That makes Syntra5 twice as effective, lowering fasting glucose by an average 107 points in just 90 days – without the kinds of dangerous side effects diabetes drugs can cause. (Of course, with major shifts like these, keeping track of your blood sugar levels is extra important.) As for the 2-hour glucose, well, the results show how incredibly Syntra5 can handle that... and in a fraction of the time of most pharmaceuticals.

Spurred by the incredibly positive results of their gold-standard clinical trial, the Syntratech team commissioned a follow-up study to see how it works and how it compared to pharmaceuticals. The subjects in this study were special type 2 diabetic mice (*Current Topics in Nutraceutical Research. Vol. 9, No. ½, 1-12, 2011*). The animals were split into 5 groups for treatment: Syntra5, Byetta, Actos, metformin, and untreated. (Byetta, Actos, and metformin are commonly prescribed diabetes drugs.)

Syntra5 was not only found to have similar actions to the diabetes drugs, it outperformed them in many crucial biomarker measurements. Most notable was Syntra5's impact on inflammation activity – and that's important because scientists have closely connected type 2 diabetes with increased inflammation. Syntra5 decreased inflammation signalling about the same as Byetta, but much more than Actos and metformin.

There are now rumours that a major east coast university in America has independently decided to study Syntra5 in a human clinical trial.

What gives Syntra5 its sugar-busting edge?

There are plenty of scientific studies backing up the sugar-busting powers of all the ingredients in Syntra5. In fact, the label reads like a 'Who's Who' of proven natural diabetes remedies:

- **HCA (hydroxycitric acid)**, from garcinia cambogia extract, has been long-studied as a weight-loss supplement, largely because it works as a natural appetite suppressant, and it's also known to keep blood insulin levels in check.

- **Gymnema sylvestre extract.** This plant has been traditionally used in Ayurvedic (ancient Indian) medicine in the fight against diabetes and now modern research findings are confirming its benefits for sufferers of the disease too. One way gymnema is thought to work is by protecting the pancreas against free radical damage, allowing it to produce insulin unhindered (*Anathna R, Latha M et al. Nutrition 2004, 20 (3): 280-285*). It also helps control blood sugar and carbohydrate cravings by actually filling the sweet receptors on your taste buds and in your digestive tract so they don't get activated when you eat sugar. A two-part study at London's King's College Hospital found that fasting and postprandial blood sugar levels in diabetic subjects improved after 60 days of treatment with gymnema extract (*Phytother Res. 2010; 24 (9): 1370-1376*). The researchers also showed that isolated pancreatic beta-cells in the laboratory secreted higher levels of insulin in the presence of gymnema extract.

- **Chromium** is well-known for keeping blood sugar in check by regulating glucose levels and even reversing insulin resistance.

- **Cinnamon extract (*Cinnamomum verum*)** – Cinnamon, the dried inner bark of a tree from Sri Lanka, is a common ingredient used to flavour a variety of dishes that you probably have sitting in your kitchen spice rack. It has a history of medicinal use that goes back thousands of years. It is well-known for keeping blood sugar in check by regulating glucose levels. Cinnamon stimulates cellular receptors to respond more efficiently to insulin and helps prevent insulin resistance. A recent review of eight separate clinical trials concluded that cinnamon is effective at reducing blood sugar levels both between and after meals, and that supplementation may help reduce complications from diabetes (*J Med Food. 2011; 14 (9): 884-889*).

- **Bitter melon extract** improves glucose tolerance and lowers blood sugar, as well as reducing insulin resistance.

- **Banaba leaf extract** contains corosolic acid, which helps your body use glucose more efficiently, and helps make sure excess glucose doesn't get stored in fat cells, making it easier to lose weight.

- **Fenugreek seed.** Fenugreek contains an amino acid called 4-hydroxyisoleucine, which – according to the results of a study on mice – is able to stimulate the secretion of insulin, reduce insulin resistance, and decrease blood sugar levels (*Curr Opin Investig Drugs. 2009; 10 (4): 353-358*). In a small clinical trial from Iran, fenugreek reduced fasting blood sugar levels by 25 per cent and blood fats by 30 per cent, in patients with type 2 diabetes (*Int J Vitam Nutr Res. 2009; 79 (1): 34-39*).

- **Vanadium**. This is a rare mineral found in fish and shellfish. The biologically active form of vanadium is called vanadyl sulphate, which has been found to stabilise blood sugar levels by making cells more sensitive to the actions of insulin and assisting in the breakdown of sugar. An animal study has revealed that it can help prevent diabetes and shift excess weight (*Cheta D et al. J Cell Mol Med 2003, 7 (4): 44*).

- **Biotin.** This vitamin lowers fasting blood glucose levels in diabetes patients and reduces insulin resistance. It helps facilitate the conversion of glucose into energy in your liver.

What to take for best results

The recommended amount is two Syntra5 tablets taken three times a day, 15-20 minutes before eating. These tablets are very large – but they need to be to include all the sugar-busting powers of the formula.

Caution: If you are already taking blood sugar medication, work with your doctor while taking Syntra5. While Syntra5 does not appear to cause hypoglycaemia (based on the studies and customer feedback), medication can, and your doctor may need to adjust your dosage.

- ### How an all-natural formula developed by a leading US doctor can help keep your blood sugar in balance

When you have high blood sugar, all of your cells are constantly surrounded by blood that contains too much glucose. And while many cells can just ignore that extra sugar – keeping their internal glucose levels normal – some can't. Those cells end up with too much internal sugar, which creates reactive oxidative stress (ROS) that can bring on conditions like neuropathy and vision loss. And once these conditions set in, they're usually permanent, since there's really nothing out there that's specifically designed to take on the complications of high blood sugar.

Fortunately, an extraordinary new product – developed by leading US physician Dr. William Campbell Douglass II – offers new hope for anyone battling high blood sugar.

GlucoComplete contains three sugar-busting ingredients with more than half a century of science to back them up. Better still, this formula addresses more than just blood glucose – it also helps protect your kidneys, heart, nerves and eyes from the ravages of excess blood sugar.

Your cells can't handle sugar without thiamine

The first ingredient in the formula is Benfotiamine – a special form of thiamine (also known as vitamin B1). It plays a key part in carbohydrate metabolism within every cell of your body, and that's the process that helps your cells handle sugar.

If you don't get enough thiamine, your cells may be literally soaking in a toxic glucose bath, giving the sugar plenty of opportunity to move in and cause all sorts of problems.

When you give your cells enough thiamine, it helps them restore their metabolic balance, which has the potential to protect your kidneys, eyes, and nerves from the oxidative damage that can be brought on by high blood sugar levels.

Are diabetic complications due to a vitamin B1 deficiency?

Pharmacist Dr. Stuart Lindsey is a type 2 diabetes sufferer who believes that many of the complications of diabetes are down to vitamin deficiencies caused by the disease and that their symptoms can be better helped by simple vitamin supplements than by drugs. His findings have just been published in the *Journal of Orthomolecular Medicine* (*J Orthomolecular Med. 2012; 27 (1): 5-8*).

Dr. Lindsey was a high street pharmacist for fifteen years, during which time he saw many people with diabetes getting onto what he calls the "sugar-med treadmill". After prolonged treatment with their diabetic medications, the health of these patients did not improve. This disturbed him. Then, pain in his feet led to his being given a diagnosis of type 2 diabetes himself, which prompted him to take a hard look at conventional assumptions and treatment.

High levels of sugar in the blood are damaging and diabetes drugs aim to correct them by driving more sugar into the cells. But exactly what damage does high blood sugar do? It appears that one of its effects is to stimulate the kidneys to excrete vitamin B1 (thiamine) at a much higher rate than normal, leading to an acute deficiency of this vitamin.

The breakthrough research that never made the news

In 2005, researcher Paul Thornalley, at the University of Essex, wrote a paper showing that many diabetic symptoms and complications may be due to a deficiency of thiamine (*Curr Diabetes Rev. 2005; 1 (3): 287-298*). Interestingly, one of the symptoms of beriberi, the classic thiamine deficiency disease, is nerve damage that looks very similar to diabetic neuropathy.

Other studies have found that deficiencies in all B-group vitamins, as well as vitamins C and D, are common in diabetics (*Brighthope IE. The Vitamin Cure for Diabetes: Prevent and treat diabetes using nutrition and vitamin supplementation. 2012 Basic Health Publications. ISBN-13: 978-1591202905*). These deficiencies can cause most of the symptoms of type 2 diabetes, including neuropathy, nephropathy (kidney damage), retinopathy (eye damage) and eventually heart failure.

Despite dire warnings from his GP, Dr. Lindsey refused to go down the drugs route and instead started to treat himself with high doses of B-vitamins and other nutrients. Within a week, the shooting pains in his ankles were mostly gone. After three weeks, all of the other symptoms of numbness of the toes and overall pain of the feet, including the 'boot effect' (the feeling that you have your boots or socks on), had also virtually disappeared.

Two years later, despite still having blood sugar readings that are considered high and for which most doctors would prescribe medication, he is free from neuropathy and has no signs of eye or kidney problems or heart disease. In his article, Dr. Lindsey says: "If all diabetics would supplement with B vitamins and vitamins C, D, and E, and minerals such as calcium and magnesium, they would lessen their problems with insulin and blood sugar, and the other serious symptoms of diabetes."

The problem with virtually all thiamine supplements is that they are water-soluble, so your body breaks them down too fast and they pass through too quickly to really help. Fortunately, benfotiamine is fat soluble, meaning it's much better absorbed by your body – up to five times more than typical thiamine supplements *(Int J Clin Pharmacol Ther. 34 (2): 47-50, 1996).*

That gives benfotiamine more time to work with your cells, helping them manage glucose much more effectively. Benfotiamine appears to act by allowing thiamine to boost the activity of an enzyme called transketolase, which helps your cells use up glucose properly *(Nature Medicine. 9 (3): 294-299, 2003).*

When transketolase levels go up, your cells have an easier time handling excess glucose. Researchers also believe that by increasing transketolase activity, benfotiamine could help protect your kidneys, eyes, nerves and heart by redirecting glucose away from damaging pathways. It may even be able to help repair your cells *(Nature Medicine. 9 (3): 294-299, 2003).*

Study after study shows just how protective benfotiamine can be

Benfotiamine appears to stop sugar-induced oxidative damage in its tracks by calming the harmful effects of elevated glucose levels (*Pharmacol Res 2010; 61 (6): 482-488; Acta Diabetol 2008; 45(3):131-141*). Specifically, in vitro studies have shown that this nutrient may actually protect endothelial cells (special cells that line the inside of blood vessels) from the effects of high blood sugar (*Diabetes 2006; 55: 2231-2237*). That's important because those special cells play a part in forming healthy blood vessels.

Not only that but an in vitro study has also found that benfotiamine may help keep cells of the retina (a critical part of eyesight) from dying off after exposure to high blood glucose levels (*Diabetes Metab Res Rev 2004; 20 (4): 330-336; Diabetes Metab Res Rev 2009; 25 (7): 647-656*).

An animal study found that three potential damage-causing biochemical pathways, which are activated by elevated blood sugar levels, had been 'normalized' in benfotiamine-treated lab rats. This was most clear in the animals' eyes; their retinas were similar to normal retinas (*Nature Medicine. 9 (3): 294-299, 2003*). Benfotiamine has also been found to exert antioxidant properties in kidney cells, also common casualties of high blood sugar (*Diabetes Metab Res Rev 2008; 24 (5): 371-377*).

It can also benefit heart health, which also needs protection from spikes in glucose levels (*Circ Heart Fail 2010; 3(2): 294-305; Circ Heart Fail 2010; 3 (2): 294-305*). Researchers found that benfotiamine helped reduce oxidative stress and helped maintain proper calcium levels in the hearts of mice – the heart can't beat properly when calcium levels aren't well-regulated (*J Appl Phyiol 2006; 100: 150-156*).

While benfotiamine helps protect many vital organs by halting oxidative stress and inflammation caused by excess glucose, what it doesn't seem to do is actually lower blood glucose levels. This brings us to the second critical ingredient in Dr. Douglass' GlucoComplete formula: Cinnamon.

Cinnamon increases insulin activity by 2,000% to keep blood sugar levels under tight control

One of the most important things cinnamon does is help your body use its own insulin to manage blood sugar more effectively, and it does that in two ways. First, unique compounds called type-A polymers boost in vitro insulin activity 20 times – that's 2,000 per cent! (*J Agric Food Chem 2004; 52 (1): 65-70*).

An animal study has also revealed that cinnamon extract is able to increase the sensitivity of the cell receptors that handle sugar metabolism by up to 33 per cent, thereby helping to improve the way glucose is handled in the body (*Diabetes Res Clin Pract 2003; 62 (3): 139-148*).

Clinical trials involving diabetic patients and cinnamon have revealed startling results

A randomized, placebo-controlled human study uncovered even more benefits (*Diabetes Care 2003; 26 (12): 3215-3218*). This 60-day trial, which included 60 subjects divided into six different treatment groups (who were also asked to modify their diets), found that the subjects in the cinnamon groups saw healthier cholesterol and triglyceride (blood fat) levels. On top of that, the people in the cinnamon groups saw substantial improvements in their fasting blood sugar levels – decreases of between 18 per cent and 29 per cent.

This trial was carried out in Pakistan and the patients' diabetes was not under the degree of control that would be typically aimed for in the West, so their blood sugar levels at the start of the trial were relatively high by comparison. The patients' diets and genetic backgrounds were also different from those of most westerners. Because of this, it was still not certain that cinnamon would be an effective addition to conventional medical treatments for diabetes.

Now, cutting-edge research from Germany has removed any remaining doubts about cinnamon's effectiveness. A team at the University of Hannover conducted a double-blind clinical trial in which 79 patients with type 2 diabetes were given either an aqueous cinnamon extract (equivalent to 3 grams of powdered cinnamon) or a placebo capsule, three times a day for four months (*Eur J Clin Invest 2006; 36 (5): 340-344*).

At the end of the trial, blood sugar levels had fallen by an average of 10 per cent in the group taking cinnamon extract, but by only 3 per cent in the control group. The patients who had the highest blood sugar readings at the start of the trial experienced the greatest reductions. This explains why the results of the German trial, while being comparable with the effects of conventional medication, were not as spectacular as those in Pakistan, where patients were starting from much higher blood sugar level readings.

Cinnulin PF lowers fasting blood sugar levels... and much more

Cinnulin PF is a special proprietary cinnamon extract that has been shown to have a very powerful effect on blood sugar: boosting glucose metabolism to significantly decrease glucose levels, along with some other very beneficial effects – and that's why Dr. Douglass decided to include this unique cinnamon extract in his formula.

In one small 12-week human trial, researchers discovered that for more than 80 per cent of the subjects, a 500mg daily dose of Cinnulin PF reduced fasting blood sugar levels by 8.4 per cent, a very substantial decrease (*J Int Soc Sports Nutr 2006; 345-53*). The subjects in the Cinnulin PF group also saw a 3.8 per cent decrease in systolic blood pressure and an improvement in their body composition – less overall body fat.

Chromium – the final ingredient in Dr. Douglass' formula

Scientists have known since the 1950s that chromium improves blood sugar management. In fact, your body can't make a substance called 'glucose tolerance factor' – which helps your body manage glucose properly – without it.

The most power comes from the chromium picolinate form – so, of course, that's the form Dr. Douglass added to GlucoComplete:

- Chromium not only increases the number of insulin receptors in the body, it also improves their performance (*J Am Coll Nutr 1998; 17 (6): 548-555*).

- A 2010 placebo-controlled human study found that 46 per cent of subjects in the chromium picolinate group (taking 1,000mcg daily for 24 weeks) showed "improved insulin sensitivity" (*Met Clin Exp 2010; 59: 755-762*).

- A 1998 review found that chromium boosted glucose tolerance in nine studies and promoted healthy cholesterol levels in five studies (*J Am Coll Nutr 1998; 17(6): 548-555*).

- A 2005 animal study found that chromium picolinate appeared to promote healthy kidney function in mice with elevated blood sugar levels (*Biol Trace Elem Res. 105 (1-3): 229-248, 2005*).

- Researchers saw significant reductions in blood glucose levels in one 1997 human study, using 1,000mcg of chromium daily (*Diabetes. 46: 1786-1791, 1997*).

What to take for best results

The recommended dosage for GlucoComplete is one capsule taken twice a day on an empty stomach (about 30 minutes before meals). It is important to inform your doctor prior to taking the formula and to have regular check-ups to assess your blood sugar levels, as the dosage of your prescription medication may need to be adjusted accordingly.

- **Discover the cutting-edge, all-natural diabetes breakthrough with a seemingly endless list of beneficial ingredients**

A brand new product called Diabet-Eze looks set to be a serious competitor to conventional diabetes drugs.

Diabet-Eze contains a remarkable 31 active nutrients and herbs, each of which plays a specific role in diabetic health. For instance, some encourage insulin secretion and regeneration of the insulin-producing cells in the pancreas, while others improve glucose uptake and blood sugar control and yet others help reduce the risk of diabetic complications.

To tell you all about the incredible anti-diabetes effects of each of the individual ingredients in Diabet-Eze would take up a whole book, so below is just a flavour of the documented benefits of eight of its most active compounds.

Chromium, calcium and magnesium are 'magic minerals' for diabetes

Chromium is a trace element that is essential for normal carbohydrate and fat metabolism. In fact, insulin simply cannot work properly without it. Studies show that people with type 2 diabetes have lower blood levels of chromium than those without the disease (*Diabetes Educ. 2004; Suppl: 2-14*). Clinical trials have demonstrated that chromium supplements enhance the metabolic action of insulin and that this effect is seen more strongly in patients whose diabetes is less well controlled (*Curr Diab Rep 2010; 10 (2): 145-151*).

Calcium is best known for keeping bones strong, but it actually has many other roles in the body. A recent study involving more than 8,000 people showed that those with the most calcium in their diets had the lowest risk of developing metabolic syndrome (a pre-diabetic condition) (*Am J Clin Nutr 2012; 95 (1): 231-40*). In a placebo-controlled trial involving 20 non-diabetic patients with high blood pressure, a supplement of 1,500mg of calcium per day for eight weeks was found to improve insulin sensitivity (*Hypertension 1997; 29: 531–536*).

Magnesium also plays a significant role in maintaining insulin sensitivity. A review published last year concluded that higher magnesium intake reduces the incidence of type 2 diabetes (*Diabetes Care 2011; 34: 2116-2122*). Diabetes disrupts magnesium metabolism, causing more to be expelled in the urine and a new clinical study has found that people with type 2 diabetes have significantly lower levels of magnesium than non-diabetic subjects (*PLoS One 2012; 7(1): e30599*).

Herbal ingredients in Diabet-Eze could be more effective than drugs

Diabet-Eze also contains a wide range of herbal extracts and phytonutrients that have been shown to help manage diabetes. Bitter melon (*Mormodica charantia*) has been found to improve insulin sensitivity, reduce blood sugar levels and suppress appetite. A clinical trial, in which researchers compared the effects in diabetes patients of a bitter melon extract and the now-banned drug Avandia (*rosiglitazone*), showed that bitter melon could be more effective in the management of diabetes and its related complications (*Phytomedicine. 2009; 16 (5): 401-405*).

Gymnema (*Gymnema sylvestre*) has been used for hundreds of years in India to treat diabetes. A two-part study at London's King's College Hospital found that fasting and postprandial blood sugar levels in diabetes patients improved after 60 days of treatment with gymnema extract (*Phytother Res. 2010; 24 (9): 1370-1376*). The researchers also showed that isolated pancreatic beta-cells (the cells that produce insulin) secreted higher levels of insulin in the presence of gymnema extract.

The Indian Kino Tree (*Pterocarpus marsupium*) is another traditional Indian treatment for diabetes. An extract of the bark has been shown to have a regenerative effect on the pancreatic beta-cells (*India J Pharmacol.*

1980; 12: 123-127). In animal experiments, an extract of the hardwood had potent anti-diabetic effects, by both stimulating insulin production and acting in the same way as insulin in allowing glucose to enter muscle cells (*J Ethnopharmacol. 2012; 141 (1): 72-79*).

Myricetin is a naturally-occurring flavonoid found in berries, fruits, vegetables, herbs, tea and wine. In experiments using obese, diabetic rats, myricetin has been found to improve the sensitivity of muscle cells to the action of insulin and to mimic the effects of insulin by stimulating glucose uptake (*J Ethnopharmacol. 2012; 141 (1): 72-79*). It has also been shown to protect the pancreatic beta-cells from the toxic effects of type 2 diabetes (*Open Biochem J. 2012; 6: 66-70*).

Diabet-Eze also contains specific anti-diabetic nutrients, such as alpha lipoic acid (ALA), which recent research has shown to be an effective alternative to conventional drugs for the management of diabetes. In a clinical trial, patients with type 2 diabetes were given varying doses of ALA (300, 600, 900, and 1,200mg/day) or placebo for 6 months and were tested for blood sugar levels and oxidative biomarkers throughout the study (*Asia Pac J Clin Nutr. 2012; 21 (1): 12-21*). The results showed that fasting blood glucose and HbA1c (glycosylated haemoglobin, an indication of long-term blood sugar levels) decreased in a dose-dependent manner in the group taking ALA.

Other important ingredients in the formula include niacin, biotin, zinc, selenium, copper, manganese, molybdenum, tungsten, rutin, luteolin, inositol, quercetin, betaine, bromelain and extracts of milk thistle, banaba leaf, green tea, valerian and black cumin seed. This incredible combination of herbs and nutrients works synergistically to maximise its anti-diabetes effects.

What to take for best results

The recommended starting dose of Diabet-Eze is six enteric-coated tablets a day (two with each meal), reducing to a maintenance dose of four tablets a day after two or three months.

It is important that you consult your doctor before using Diabet-Eze, especially if you are currently on any medication. Your blood sugar levels will need to be closely monitored by your doctor and the dosage of your medication may need to be adjusted accordingly.

Because the luteolin used in Diabet-Eze is derived from peanut shells, this product is not recommended for people with a peanut allergy.

• Medicinal mushrooms can aid blood sugar control

In the Far East, mushrooms have been used for centuries for their powerful medicinal properties. Recent research has shown that some kinds of mushrooms contain compounds that can help to control blood sugar levels.

In 2011, two detailed scientific reviews were published on the use of mushrooms for the prevention and treatment of diabetes (*Functional Foods in Health and Disease 2011; 4: 161-171; Int J Med Mushrooms. 2011; 13 (5): 401-26*). What these reviews revealed was that mushrooms contain many different chemicals that can aid blood sugar control, through a variety of biological mechanisms in the body.

Some of these natural anti-diabetes compounds inhibit the absorption of glucose, others protect the insulin-producing beta-cells in the pancreas from damage or increase the amount of insulin released, while yet others regulate complex processes called insulin signalling pathways, by which glucose is absorbed from the bloodstream into muscle, fat or brain cells.

Several of these individual compounds have been isolated, extracted and patented by pharmaceutical companies for use as medicines. This is not because they work better in isolation from the whole mushrooms, but because the pharmaceutical companies can make a lot of money out of them that way!

One reason why mushrooms are so effective in helping to control blood sugar is their content of beta-glucans. These are part of a family of chemicals called polysaccharides, which also includes cellulose, the material from which the cell walls of most plants is constructed. The cell walls of mushrooms, on the other hand, are made of beta-glucans and these differ slightly in their chemical structure between different species of mushrooms.

These small differences are important, since not all beta-glucans are equal when it comes to blood sugar control. The most effective ones are found in the mushrooms that have been traditionally used in Chinese medicine, such as shiitake, maitake, reishi, coriolus, cordiceps and agaricus. Beta-glucans extracted from yeast or barley, which are cheaper to produce, do not have such strong effects on human biology.

Beta-glucans reduce the glycaemic index of a meal

In a clinical trial carried out by the Functional Food Centre at Oxford Brookes University, spaghetti that was enriched with beta-glucans was found to have a glycaemic index of less than half that of normal spaghetti, which was used as a control (*Nutrition. 2011; 27 (6): 653-658*). That is to say, the beta-glucan enriched spaghetti had less than half the impact on blood sugar levels. The scientists used beta-glucans derived from barley in this trial and it is likely that mushroom beta glucans have an even stronger effect in moderating the rise in blood sugar after a meal.

Animal tests have shown just how effective medicinal mushrooms can be in combating high blood sugar levels, although large-scale clinical trials in humans are still needed to verify these results. Medicinal mushrooms contain many other blood sugar-regulating compounds in addition to beta-glucans. Researchers in Korea found that an extract of the mushroom Agaricus blazei, from which the beta-glucans had been removed, reduced blood sugar levels in diabetic rats as effectively as the standard diabetes drug metformin (*J Agric Food Chem. 2010; 58 (7): 4113-4119*).

Other animal trials have found a range of medicinal mushrooms, particularly Cordyceps militaris, to be very effective in reducing blood sugar levels (*Appl Microbiol Biotechnol. 2006; 72 (6): 1152-1156*).

One of the best ways to benefit from these amazingly beneficial plants, which have also been shown to support the immune system and protect against heart disease and cancer, is to take a supplement. There are a number of single and combination mushroom products available.

- ## This incredible Chinese mushroom could slash your risk of diabetes, heart disease and cancer

Red reishi (*Ganoderma lucidum*) has long been considered the number one herb in traditional Chinese medicine and is known as the 'mushroom of immortality'. In fact, it was once reserved solely for the use of emperors, who believed it would grant them eternal youth and good health.

After centuries of anecdotal evidence and hundreds of research papers, placebo-controlled clinical trials have now proved reishi's amazing ability to boost the immune system and even fight certain cancers (*Chem Biodivers 2007; 4 (2): 224-231; Perspectives in Biology and Medicine 2006; 49 (2): 159-170*). Other studies also suggest its potential benefits in health problems as diverse as diabetes, heart disease, prostate enlargement and chronic fatigue.

Red reishi is generally considered to be the most potent variety of the reishi mushroom. One of the highest quality supplements on the market is Mikei Red Reishi Essence. Red reishi's effectiveness largely depends on the conditions in which it is cultivated. The mushrooms for Mikei Red Reishi Essence are grown on carefully selected Japanese aged oak logs, producing one of the most superior red reishi extracts available. More than 200 different substances have been isolated from red reishi, among which polysaccharides and triterpenoids have been identified as the main groups of active components.

Studies indicate that various polysaccharides are responsible for strengthening and modulating the immune system, whereas triterpenoids (of which more than 119 have already been found in red reishi) have direct anti-tumour and anti-inflammatory effects (*Planta Med 2009, 25*

Aug [Epub ahead of print]). Red reishi's other ingredients may also work synergistically to contribute to its disease-fighting effects.

Red reishi reduces blood sugar levels

An animal study carried out at the University of Hong Kong has shown that red reishi could be valuable in the management of diabetes and metabolic syndrome. Red reishi was found to switch off a gene responsible for the production of glucose in the liver and in doing so, reduced blood sugar levels (*Phytomedicine 2009; 16(5): 426-436*). Interestingly, this is exactly the same mechanism by which the diabetes drug metformin works.

A separate study with rats has found that red reishi extract protects the insulin-producing cells in the pancreas from experimentally-induced damage by alloxan, a chemical that selectively destroys these cells (*Life Sci 2003; 73 (18): 2307-2319*).

Red reishi also has a reputation for maintaining a healthy heart and circulation, which is important for diabetics. Research shows it reduces both blood pressure and the levels of fats in the blood (*J Nutr Sci Vitaminol (Tokyo) 1988; 34 (4): 433-438*). Animal studies carried out in Taiwan have revealed that red reishi's antioxidant properties can protect the heart from free radical damage (*Phytother Res 2004; 18(12): 1024-1026*). What's more, recent work by Russian scientists suggests that red reishi could prevent damage to heart tissue during a heart attack (*Patol Fiziol Eksp Ter 2008; 1: 22-25*).

In addition to all these health benefits, red reishi is an adaptogen – a substance that helps the body to deal with stress – and it is often used to aid restful sleep. In today's hectic world, with so much to worry us, red reishi could be an ancient remedy with a thoroughly modern application.

What to take for best results

Mikei Red Reishi Essence comes in packs of 30 capsules, each containing

250mg of concentrated red reishi essence powder. The recommended dosage is one capsule a day. Women who are pregnant or breastfeeding are advised to consult their doctor before taking Mikei Red Reishi Essence.

- **Discover the all-natural formula that helps prevent diabetic complications and the ageing effects of high blood sugar**

We all know that sugar is bad for us. When we eat more than we can burn off as energy, the excess is converted to fat, leading to weight gain. That is bad enough, but there is another, even more sinister side to sugar. When there is more sugar in your body than you need (and this can come from the breakdown of starchy carbohydrates as well as from sugar that you eat), it reacts with proteins and fats, in a process called glycation. A whole chain of reactions is involved, ending with the formation of compounds known as 'advanced glycation end-products', or AGE.

AGE is an appropriate acronym for these sticky, damaging substances, which cause much of the deterioration and discomfort associated with premature ageing. AGE accumulate throughout the body in skin, muscle, joint, brain, and organ tissues and have been linked to a host of maladies associated with getting older. AGE weld protein molecules together in unnatural ways, called cross-linking, which rob affected tissues of movement and function. This damage makes normal, supple body structures stiff and brittle, impairs nerve function, contributes to plaque build-up in your arteries, clogs neural pathways in the brain and destroys capillaries in the kidneys and eyes (*Diabetologia 2001; 44 (2): 129-146*).

The gradual build-up of AGE is a normal part of the ageing process, but it is massively accelerated by a high-carbohydrate diet and by a shortage of certain nutrients. Unfortunately, AGE cannot be broken down any further and usually remain in the body forever. Because they cannot be dissolved or eliminated, the only way to prevent the adverse effects of AGE is to block their formation.

Now there is an easy and effective way that you can slow down the formation of AGE and limit the effect of these harmful molecules. Lypo-Spheric AGE Blocker, from LivOn Laboratories, contains a unique formulation of B vitamins, trace minerals, antioxidants and cinnamon extract, designed for the very purpose of intercepting sugar metabolism by-products before they can be converted to AGE. Benfotiamine (a vitamin B1 derivative), pyridoxal and pyridoxamine (forms of vitamin B6), for example, are known to block AGE formation (*Exp Gerontol 2011; 46 (6): 482-488*).

Not only that but the other B vitamins, trace minerals and cinnamon extract work together to help facilitate proper glucose metabolism, lower insulin resistance, and improve energy levels.

A technological breakthrough helps guarantee that the beneficial ingredients are properly absorbed

As well as containing a host of beneficial nutrients, Lypo-Spheric AGE Blocker delivers them reliably into your bloodstream using a patented technology that increases their bioavailability enormously.

For years, researchers have known about the 'gastro-intestinal barrier', which restricts the amount of nutrients you can absorb from your gut at any one time. This has been a major problem for food supplement manufacturers because they know that, with normal product formulations, only a small proportion of the content is actually going to be absorbed.

LivOn's patented liposomal encapsulation technology has overcome this problem by creating 'smart' Lyposomal Nano-Spheres, which are microscopic bubbles of essential phospholipids. These provide an oral delivery system that can carry almost 100 per cent of any nutrient through the gastro-intestinal barrier and get it to where it is needed in the body. In addition, each dose of Lypo-Spheric AGE Blocker is sealed in its own package, to protect it from light and oxygen and so guarantee its freshness and potency.

The results of a new clinical trial from India demonstrate the ability of AGE-blocking nutrients to improve endothelial dysfunction (an early stage in hardening of the arteries) in patients with rheumatoid arthritis (*Int J Rheum Dis 2012; 15 (1): 45-55*). The trial involved 24 patients with high levels of inflammatory activity, a contributory factor in endothelial dysfunction, despite treatment with conventional drugs. Taking 50mg of benfotiamine, 50mg of pyridoxamine and 500 micrograms of methylcobalamin (a form of vitamin B12 that is also an ingredient of Lypo-Spheric AGE Blocker) twice a day for 12 weeks resulted in greater flexibility and dilation of the arteries and significantly reduced markers for inflammation in the blood.

Lypo-Spheric AGE Blocker could help you to avoid diabetic retinopathy and neuropathy

Because people with diabetes or metabolic syndrome tend to have elevated levels of blood sugar, they are at increased risk of producing AGE at an accelerated rate. Diabetic retinopathy, a complication of diabetes involving damage to blood vessels in the retina of the eye, may be one result of increased AGE formation (*Amino Acids 2012; 42 (4): 1163-70*).

Researchers have also established an association between AGE and diabetic neuropathy, a type of nerve damage that causes numbness or pain in the hands, feet, arms or legs. In animal experiments, benfotiamine and pyridoxamine both proved effective in improving this condition, although equivalent effects have yet to be established in human clinical trials (*Ann N Y Acad Sci 2005; 1043: 784-792*).

In addition to the potent AGE inhibitors benfotiamine and pyridoxamine, Lypo-Spheric AGE Blocker also contains the full range of B-complex vitamins and related nutrients, including B2 (riboflavin), B3 (niacin), B6 (as pyridoxal-5-phosphate), B12, biotin and folic acid. These nutrients are an integral part of the body's glucose metabolism and energy production and are frequently lacking in the typical British diet.

A wide range of trace minerals is included in Lypo-Spheric AGE Blocker, for their properties in aiding correct glucose metabolism and in counteracting the effects of ageing. These include chromium, magnesium, boron, indium, manganese, selenium, vanadium and zinc. Cinnamon extract is also an ingredient as it has been shown to be helpful in controlling blood sugar levels. A recent meta-analysis of eight separate clinical studies concluded that cinnamon (powder or extract) improves fasting blood glucose in people with type 2 diabetes or pre-diabetes *(J Med Food 2011; 14 (9): 884-889)*.

What to take for best results

The recommended dose of Lypo-Spheric AGE Blocker is one or two sachets per day. For best results, the contents of the sachet should be stirred into a cool drink and taken on an empty stomach (15 to 20 minutes before a meal if you suffer with symptoms of low blood sugar). The product should not be mixed with a hot beverage or used with a blender or food processor.

- ### Ivy gourd heralds a long awaited breakthrough in the fight against diabetes

Ivy gourd (also known as *Coccinia indica*, *Coccinia cordifolia* and *Coccinia grandis*) is a creeping plant – a tropical flowering vine that grows abundantly in Hawaii, India and other Southeast Asian countries such as Thailand and Indonesia.

While in Hawaii it's considered invasive – a reputation that has prompted the label 'noxious weed' – in other countries it's highly esteemed. Natives to India embrace the vine's fruit as a common staple in the kitchen, using it in curries and soups, stuffing it with masala or simply frying it. But that's not all – the leaves and shoots of this plant are edible too. And it's a good thing, because as super foods go, they don't get much more powerful than this.

In recent years, studies have revealed something that Ayurvedic practitioners have known for centuries, that ivy gourd is one of the most potent natural diabetes treatments out there. Several animal studies have shown that this herb has some pretty remarkable hypoglycaemic benefits, with particularly positive results in cases of type 2 diabetes (*Indian J Med Sci. 1998 Apr; 52 (4): 143-6; Ethnopharmacol. 2003 Jan; 84 (1): 105-8*).

What's even more exciting, though, is that these results extend to human studies, too. These extremely promising findings have led researchers, including those at the prestigious Harvard Medical School, to place ivy gourd in a class by itself. Stacked up against a cornucopia of well-known anti-diabetic herbs, this natural dynamo has the best clinical evidence backing it up by far *(Diabetes Care. 2003 Apr; 26 (4): 1277-94)*.

Compounds in this plant inhibit the enzyme glucose-6-phosphatase, which is one of the key liver enzymes involved in regulating sugar metabolism. In a double-blind trial, 60 patients with newly-diagnosed type 2 diabetes were given an ivy gourd extract or placebo for 90 days (*Diabetes Care. 2008; 31 (2): 216-220*). When tested, the ivy gourd group had fasting blood sugar levels that were 16 per cent lower than those of the placebo group and postprandial (after meal) levels that were 18 per cent lower.

More research is needed to shed light on the true scope of this herb's potential. And for now, at least, it seems to remain a secret under the natural health industry's radar – outside of its native India, that is.

- **Discover the ancient herb that is causing a real stir in scientific circles for its ability to take on diabetes, high blood pressure and fatigue**

Sun Eleuthero is a top quality herbal preparation from the roots of the *Eleutherococcus senticosus* plant, also known as Siberian ginseng. In the last decade, research into this powerful herb has gathered an astonishing pace, revealing a diverse range of therapeutic properties and giving new hope to sufferers of diabetes, chronic fatigue, high blood pressure and even degenerative conditions like Alzheimer's and Parkinson's.

Famed as an energy tonic in China for more than 2,000 years, the benefits of Eleutherococcus only gained recognition in the West in the 1950s, when Russian scientists reported on its amazing stress-lowering action. People taking the herb were found to better endure physical strain, resist disease, and perform tests of mental sharpness. In a further series of landmark Russian studies in the 1960s, healthy adults given Eleutherococcus experienced increased stamina for physical tasks, withstood motion sickness better and were able to work with speed and precision despite being surrounded by loud noise.

Because this herb appeared to the Russian researchers to have similar effects to those of Korean ginseng (*Panax ginseng*), it was promoted and marketed as 'Siberian ginseng', despite the fact that the two plants are only distantly related botanically. More lately, it has become referred to as 'eleuthero', particularly in the US, in order to avoid any confusion with true ginseng. Far from being ginseng's poor relative, though, eleuthero has a wealth of unique health-promoting properties, many of which have only recently become apparent following a series of studies.

In developing Sun Eleuthero, the Sun Chlorella Corporation was determined to use the best quality roots from genuine eleuthero plants, which grow naturally only in the wild, unpolluted areas of Northeast Asia and Northeast Hokkaido (the most northerly island of Japan). This is important because a 2008 study using DNA analysis revealed that herbal medicines sold as eleuthero in China and Japan are made from at least three different plants, and only around 70 per cent of them contain the correct species *(Planta Med 2008; 74 (7): 787-789)*.

New studies reveal how eleuthero helps regulate blood sugar

If the results of animal studies can be replicated in humans, then eleuthero may prove beneficial for people with diabetes or insulin resistance. Animal studies have revealed that it helps keep blood sugar levels stable. Doctors at Taipei Medical University in Taiwan found that blood sugar levels in diabetic rats dropped significantly 30 minutes after they were injected with syringin, one of the main active ingredients in *Eleutherococcus senticosus* extract (*Horm Metab Res 2007; 39 (12): 894-898*).

Syringin helps boost the secretion of a neurotransmitter chemical in the brain called beta-endorphin, which in turn stimulates the sympathetic nervous system, resulting in a fall in blood sugar levels. In further studies with non-diabetic rats, the same researchers found that syringin reduced the hike in blood sugar following a glucose injection, due to its ability to promote the uptake of glucose by muscle cells (*Planta Med 2008; 74 (2): 109-113*).

Of course, the results of animal studies, particularly where active ingredients are injected, may not automatically apply to people taking a herbal extract as a food supplement. However, the results of these studies lend weight to the traditional use of eleuthero to help control diabetes.

Eleuthero may also help to reduce high blood pressure by relaxing the walls of blood vessels, according to studies carried out by researchers at McMaster University in Ontario, Canada (*Naunyn Schmiedebergs Arch Pharmacol 2004; 369 (5): 473-480*).

In addition, South Korean scientists have discovered that rats injected with an extract of the herb had much less brain damage from artificially-induced strokes than controls (*Phytother Res 2005; 19 (2): 167-169*). This effect seems to be due to eleuthero's ability to inhibit the activation of microglia, a type of immune cell specific to the brain. Activated microglia produce various inflammatory substances and are implicated in both Alzheimer's disease and Parkinson's disease.

What to take for best results

Sun Eleuthero comes as very small tablets, in packs of 300 or 1,500. It is recommended to start with 5 tablets a day and work up to a daily dosage of 15 tablets. It is best taken in the morning before food, but can be spread throughout the day if preferred. Sun Eleuthero is also available as a liquid extract and as a tea.

Diabetics should talk to their doctor before starting Sun Eleuthero, particularly if they are taking prescription medication.

- ## A new supplement heralds good news for sufferers of diabetes and cancer

Scientists have known for some time now that a naturally-occurring substance, found in your body's cells and also present in vegetable fibre, is an effective anti-cancer agent. Now, there is mounting evidence to suggest that this active compound could also play a vital role in the prevention and management of type 2 diabetes.

Inositol hexaphosphate (IP6), also known as phytic acid, is a component of fibre found in whole grains and legumes (peas and beans). However, the quantities of IP6 derived from these dietary sources are too small to provide any real therapeutic value. Now this problem has finally been overcome following the development of IP6 in supplement form. Taken in this way, more of it can be efficiently absorbed and utilised by your body.

Following a review of numerous study results, US scientists have concluded that IP6 – and its related substance IP3 (formed when IP6 enters your body) – could be the key to regulating healthy insulin production (*Journal of Physiology Endocrinology and Metabolism, Dec. 2002, 283, p E1113-E1122*). Their findings open exciting doors to the future management of diabetes and herald a brighter future for those with a family history of the disease who are trying to prevent its onset in later life.

How cancer research led to this exciting discovery

Naturopath Marcus Webb, who also works as a chartered biologist and technical director at Hadley Wood Healthcare, the company behind the development of IP6, says that the excitement about IP6 and diabetes has come about almost as a 'side effect' of the extensive research into IP6 and cancer.

In fact, over the past 15 years, studies on IP6 have mainly focused on its role as an antioxidant and anti-cancer agent. A leader in this field has been Dr. Abul Shamsuddin, Professor of Medicine at the University of Maryland School of Medicine, in Baltimore in the US. He and fellow researchers have published a number of key papers on the benefits of IP6 in fighting cancer.

One of the reasons why it is thought to be so effective in this area is due to the fact that it is a powerful antioxidant – meaning that it helps render free radicals harmless, which can otherwise increase the risk of the disease developing. According to scientists IP6 may also help to inhibit the spread of established cancer, as it has been shown to slow down the rate of abnormal cell division (*International Journal of Food Science and Technology, 2002, Vol 37, p 769-782; I Vucenik, AM Shamsuddin. Inhibition of growth and induction of differentiation by IP6. June 2002. European Cancer Research Symposium, Granada, Spain*).

It also boosts immunity by increasing the activity of natural killer cells, which help fight off viruses, bacteria and cancerous cells. Not only that but it may also have the added benefit of preventing the formation of kidney stones (*F Grases, BM Simonet, I Vucenik, J Perello, RM Prieto, AM Shamsuddin. Effects of exogenous inositol hexaphosphate (InsP6) on the levels of InsP6 and of inositol trisphosphate (InsP3) in malignant cells, tissues and biological fluids. Laboratory of Renal Lithiasis Research, Faculty of Science, University of Balearic Islands, Palma de Mallorca, Spain, Life Sciences, 16 August 2002, p 1535-1546).*

Marcus Webb says that in the course of patients taking IP6 for the above medical complaints, researchers noticed that many of them were not only experiencing health-related benefits in these specific areas, but tests were also revealing healthier blood sugar levels.

According to Marcus, IP6 probably helps to benefit health in so many different ways because it appears to play a key role in cell-to-cell communication. He says: "The anecdotal evidence is supported by a good grounding in the theory of how it should work"... "And the more you look into the cellular basis of disease, the more you see that communication between cells is at the roots of it".

"Since I've been taking it, I feel better and I feel fitter... and my blood sugar level has come down"

When IP6 enters the body it divides to produce two molecules of IP3; it is IP3 that plays a major role in the communication between cells. In this new IP6 supplement, IP6 is combined in a four-to-one ratio with inositol (a member of the B-vitamin group), which helps IP6 to create IP3 more efficiently.

IP6 and IP3 help regulate blood sugar levels by encouraging the efficient functioning of beta cells in your pancreas. Scientists know that these cells are sensitive to glucose and are responsible for the process that leads to insulin (which helps regulate glucose) being released. If these cells are not working properly then type 2 diabetes can occur.

One person to benefit from taking IP6 supplements is well-known TV personality, naturopath and health expert, Jan De Vries. He has been taking them for the past four months to help manage his type 2 diabetes, and he says he has already noticed "a distinct improvement" in his condition.

Jan De Vries is sure that IP6 also gives the body's immune system a boost, and says, "since I've been taking it, I feel better and I feel fitter... and my blood sugar level has come down." He has just completed work on a new book entitled *My Life With Diabetes*, in which he mentions the benefits of IP6 in helping to manage his condition.

What to take for best results

The recommended dosage is two capsules of IP6 taken twice a day. In powder form, the suggested dose is one scoop twice a day (see label for further details). There have not been any reports of side effects linked to taking IP6 supplements, but as always check with your doctor if you are currently on any medication.

- **The cactus that helps stop your blood sugar levels from soaring – lowering your risk of diabetes**

Nopal is derived from the prickly pear cactus, which is native to Mexico and the south-western regions of the US. In Mexico, its use as a food and medicine dates back to the Aztec period, 900-1521 AD. After the spines have been removed, this tasty ripe fruit has a unique sweet flavour that continues to be a staple in the Mexican diet.

Its historical uses as a medicine include being taken as a cardiac tonic. The peeled stems of the cactus were also applied directly to wounds in order to facilitate the healing process and promote a speedy recovery.

Recent studies suggest that Nopal has a valuable role to play in overcoming a wide range of medical conditions. It has been found to be beneficial in helping to regulate blood sugar levels, aid weight loss, lower cholesterol levels and overcome gastrointestinal disorders like constipation.

Nopal supplements are of an extremely high quality – they are formulated using extracts from Nopal cacti that are cultivated on the slopes of the mountains of Jalisco state in Mexico. In this region the soil is particularly rich, as it is irrigated by natural spring water and remains free from harmful chemicals and fertilisers.

An abundant source of essential nutrients

It is little wonder that Nopal is able to exert so many therapeutic actions considering it is packed full of essential nutrients. It contains the vitamins: A, B1, B2, B3, and C; in addition to the minerals: potassium, calcium, magnesium and iron. Also present are 18 amino acids in the form of easily digestible protein.

As a fibrous plant, Nopal is a rich source of insoluble and soluble fibre. It is its high-fibre content that is thought to be largely responsible for so many of its healthful benefits.

Soluble fibre helps maintain normal blood sugar levels

It is the soluble fibre compounds – including mucilages, gums and pectin – that are believed to be the main reason why Nopal is so effective in helping to stabilise blood sugar levels.

Soluble fibre is associated with slowing stomach-emptying time due to its gelling properties when mixed with water – a mechanism that causes food to be absorbed into the blood stream at a much slower rate and prevents sudden surges in blood sugar.

Soluble fibre can also lower blood sugar levels in people with diabetes, and some researchers have found that increasing dietary fibre intake can decrease the body's need for insulin (*American Journal of Clinical Nutrition 1979; 32: 2312-21*).

Managing diabetes without a long-term reliance on insulin injections

In an animal study, researchers found that diabetes could be successfully controlled following the use of a purified extract of the Nopal cactus (*Journal of Ethnopharmacology 1996; 55: 27-33*). The study involved four groups of rats, three of which were diabetic, and a non-diabetic control group. The diabetic rats were given either insulin, Nopal extract, or a combination of insulin and Nopal extract.

Throughout the study, the glucose levels of the control group remained similar to initial levels. The insulin-treated diabetic rats showed high glucose levels after one week, which then decreased by week two and stabilised at moderately high levels thereafter.

The diabetic rats receiving Nopal extract were found to have glucose levels similar to those of the insulin-treated rats. The diabetic rats receiving both insulin and Nopal extract were the only group with normalised glucose levels. Within two weeks, glucose levels in this group had declined to levels found in the control group. Insulin treatment was stopped and normal glucose levels were maintained with Nopal extract alone.

The scientists concluded that the control of diabetes by purified extract of Nopal can be attained with daily oral doses in the range of 1mg/kg body weight.

Nopal may help type 2 diabetics in more ways than one

Based on a survey of South Texas residents, researchers have been assessing the link between Nopal and the metabolic control of people with type 2 diabetes (*Annu Meet Int Soc Technol Assess Health Care, 1996; 12:14*).

Although definite conclusions cannot be made until more data becomes available, preliminary findings are extremely promising and strongly suggest that Nopal may be an effective natural remedy for the successful management of type 2 diabetes.

Analysis of six medical studies from Mexico has provided evidence to show that Nopal reduces serum glucose levels in diabetics within 30 to 180 minutes after ingestion.

Another way Nopal may help in the prevention and treatment of type 2 diabetes is the area of obesity – a contributing factor in causing the condition. Nopal's ability to help promote weight loss is due to the fact that it absorbs water upon ingestion, which produces a feeling of fullness. This, combined with its positive effect on blood sugar levels, appears to help reduce appetite and control carbohydrate cravings.

Nopal can alleviate digestive problems and bring cholesterol levels down

Nopal's insoluble fibre content increases the bulk of faecal matter, which encourages regular bowel movements. Insoluble fibre helps shorten the rate of transit time through your gastro-intestinal tract, preventing the accumulation of waste materials and reducing the risk of bowel conditions such as constipation, diverticulitis (the development of abnormal, inflamed pouches in the colon) and haemorrhoids.

Another area Nopal is proving to be effective in is lowering cholesterol and triglyceride (blood fat) levels. High levels of either can substantially increase your risk of chronic conditions like heart disease.

This beneficial action is thought to be due to the soluble fibre – particularly in the form of mucilages and pectin – present in Nopal. It binds with bile acids that emulsify fats in the gut, which encourages their excretion from your body and prevents the build-up of fatty deposits on your artery walls.

What to take for best results

The recommended dosage is two capsules of Nopal taken with a glass of water before meals.

Due to the fact that Nopal has a normalising effect on blood sugar levels, diabetic patients should check with their GP before taking it – particularly as medication dosage amounts may need to be reduced.

- **The daily multivitamin supplement that can keep blood sugar levels healthy**

From what you've read in this report so far, you will be aware of the benefits of keeping your blood sugar under control. While your body can generally deal with the occasional blood sugar hike, consistently high levels can lead to weight gain, heart disease and diabetes.

Now, a new daily multivitamin and mineral supplement is available that has the added benefit of helping to keep your blood sugar levels within normal limits.

After a meal or snack, the hormone insulin, which you produce in your pancreas, pushes glucose into your muscle cells for energy production. But unless you are very careful about what you eat and drink, blood sugar levels can soar too high, leading to the over-production of insulin. This can cause a 'roller coaster' effect in which blood sugar plummets, making you crave a sugary snack, which then starts the process all over again.

Apart from making you feel alternately wired and exhausted, poor blood sugar control has a more sinister side. Too much insulin causes the liver to release large amounts of fat into the bloodstream (*J Nutrition 2001; 131: 2074*). This increases the risk of heart disease or stroke. Too much fat and sugar in the blood can also block insulin receptors on the muscle cells, leading to 'insulin resistance' and weight gain, and ultimately type 2 diabetes.

Multi-Guard Control, from British firm Lamberts, is a daily multivitamin and mineral formula that also includes ingredients to stabilise blood sugar levels.

Cinnamon controls blood sugar

Multi-Guard Control provides good amounts of 26 nutrients including, per daily dose, a full 2,000mg of cinnamon. Studies have confirmed that cinnamon has a positive effect on glucose metabolism in people with blood sugar imbalance. Tests on cinnamon have indicated that it may work by helping to activate the insulin receptors on muscle cells, increasing insulin sensitivity.

In one study of subjects with blood sugar imbalance, cinnamon lowered levels of LDL (low-density lipoprotein) and total cholesterol as well as blood sugar levels (*Diabetes Care 2003; 26: 3215-3218*). This suggests that cinnamon may additionally hold promise for helping to reduce the cardiovascular risk factors associated with blood sugar disorders.

In a US clinical trial carried out at the Wadsworth Medical Centre in Ohio, 22 subjects with pre-diabetes and insulin resistance were randomly assigned to take either cinnamon extract or a placebo for 12 weeks. Measurements were taken at the start and end of the study of their 'fasting blood glucose' (FBG – the blood sugar level in the morning before eating, which is an indicator for diabetes), blood pressure and fat to muscle ratio.

People taking the cinnamon extract had significant drops in their FBG levels and blood pressure, and increases in lean body mass, compared with the placebo group. The researchers concluded that "this naturally-occurring spice can reduce risk factors associated with diabetes and cardiovascular diseases" (*J Int Soc Sports Nutr 2006; 3: 45-53*).

Multi-Guard Control against diabetes

Multi-Guard Control also contains 200µg of GTF ('glucose tolerance factor') chromium, which is probably the best known of all the blood sugar control nutrients. Animal studies have found that GTF chromium prevents the kidney damage that can be associated with diabetes and researchers report "a remarkable decrease in plasma lipids (blood fats) and glucose from administration of GTF" (*J Am Soc Nephrol 2006; 17 (4 Suppl 2): S127-31*).

The 300mg of magnesium in Multi-Guard Control has been included because it is a component of many enzymes involved in the breakdown of blood sugar and acts as a 'secondary messenger' for the activity of insulin at the cellular membrane level. Magnesium is required for both the proper utilisation of glucose and for the prevention of insulin resistance (*Magnesium Res 2004; 17 (2): 126-136*).

There is also 150mg of alpha lipoic acid (ALA) in Multi-Guard Control, since research has shown it can activate the so-called 'insulin signalling cascade' in cells. Studies in individuals with blood sugar imbalance have shown that ALA can improve glucose uptake by enhancing insulin sensitivity.

ALA plays a role in preventing diabetes by reducing fat accumulation. In animal studies, ALA reduced body weight, protected pancreatic beta cells (the insulin producing cells) from destruction, and reduced fat accumulation in muscle tissues and the pancreas (*Biochem Biophys Res Commun. 2005 Jan 7; 326 (1): 197–202*).

ALA is also a powerful antioxidant that positively affects important aspects of diabetes, including blood sugar control and the development of long-term complications such as diseases of the heart, kidneys, small blood vessels and nerves.

Other nutrients that have also been shown to help support glucose utilisation include: zinc, vitamin C and in particular the vitamins B1, B3 and B6. These nutrients are all included at significant levels in Multi-Guard Control.

What to take for best results

Take two Multi-Guard Control tablets daily, preferably one with breakfast and the other one with either lunch or dinner. Because this product contains iron, it may be harmful to very young children, so keep it out of their sight and reach. Consult your doctor before taking this supplement if you are pregnant or breast-feeding.

- **The Chinese herbal remedy that can reverse metabolic syndrome and protect against type 2 diabetes**

As previously mentioned, metabolic syndrome isn't a disease but a group of symptoms that are linked to your body's metabolism. These symptoms include excess body fat around your abdomen, high triglyceride (blood fat) levels, elevated blood pressure, low levels of 'good' high-density lipoprotein (HDL) cholesterol, and high blood sugar levels.

If left unchecked, the onset of type 2 diabetes is a looming inevitability, as are its often-fatal complications, including heart disease, kidney failure, neuropathy and blindness. Considering the severity of these conditions, it's alarming that metabolic syndrome is so common – it's estimated that up to a quarter of people in the UK may currently be suffering from it (*British Nutrition Foundation Obesity and disease in ageing: Report 2: The metabolic syndrome Available at: http://www.nutrition.org.uk (accessed November 10, 2004)*).

Fortunately, a cutting-edge herbal remedy called MetaPhase has become available. The formula is manufactured by a US company called Tango Advanced Nutrition, although it originated in China where the herbs it contains have been found to help stabilise erratic blood sugar levels and keep type 2 diabetes at bay. It also supports organs such as the pancreas, stomach, liver and gall bladder – all of which contribute to your body's metabolic functions.

Eastern wisdom for a Western malady

After years of clinical evaluations in China, this proprietary blend of herbs was developed to treat the growing problems of insulin resistance and type 2 diabetes that accompanied the country's newly acquired Western eating habits.

The formula met with astonishing success, to the extent that one of the Chinese study participants – an insulin-dependent type 2 diabetic – was weaned off his daily injections altogether.

Impressed by the promise that MetaPhase could herald a breakthrough treatment for one of the West's most imminent – and medicated – health threats, scientists at Tango Advanced Nutrition decided to investigate the formula further. They subjected samples to a battery of tests to assure the safety and purity of each individual ingredient, as well as the product as a whole.

MetaPhase encourages your body to heal itself

The three main ingredients in MetaPhase are Lycium root-bark, turmeric and cordyceps. Lycium root-bark is the lead herb, appearing in the formula in the largest quantities, and is a modern staple in Chinese herbal diabetes treatments due to its ability to lower blood pressure and regulate blood sugar levels.

Turmeric is used in many Chinese formulas to reduce inflammation, calm the nerves, and restore gall bladder function, enhancing bile secretion and facilitating the digestion of fats. Cordyceps is also adept at reducing blood sugar and is said to have overall strengthening properties.

With these three herbs acting as MetaPhase's main players, four additional herbs assume the supporting roles:

- Barbary wolfberry is a popular Chinese health-food herb that supports the liver and kidneys, benefits vision, and replenishes energy.

- Curcubita fruit (the botanical name for pumpkin) can help reduce blood sugar levels.

- Chinese hawthorn improves blood circulation, lowers cholesterol and blood pressure, and supports proper digestion.

- Ophiopogon has traditionally been used in China to: prevent the fluid loss that results from diabetic disorders; support and restore pancreatic function; reduce blood sugar and relax the muscles.

The last ingredient, jujube seed, is a newcomer to the arena of diabetic herbal formulas. But in China, it's the main component of all addiction remedies on account of its demonstrated calming effects. For this same reason, it eases the agitation that accompanies the overwhelming cravings prompted by glucose and insulin imbalances.

Lower your blood sugar levels and recharge your batteries

While more studies are needed to confirm the product's efficacy, the testimonials attesting to its benefits certainly aren't lacking.

Take Myrna for instance... she was shocked when she received the news from her doctor at the age of 69 that her blood sugar levels were dangerously high, as prior to this she'd never experienced any major problems with her health.

But Myrna was reluctant to start popping pills to combat her blood sugar problem. As she put it, "I've never depended on medications before and I'm not about to start now." However, tackling the condition without pharmaceutical help soon began to look like wishful thinking – until Myrna's niece, a nutritionist versed in the field of alternative health, told her about MetaPhase.

Three months after taking the product her blood sugar levels dropped significantly, and, according to Myrna, she feels like she did 10 years ago. Her energy has skyrocketed, allowing her to function on eight hours of sleep instead of her usual 11. She even lost a little bit of weight, mostly around her waist – something that, until now, defied even her best efforts. Better still, she had achieved these results while only taking the maintenance dosage – less than half of what is initially recommended.

MetaPhase can put a stop to persistent cravings once and for all

Paul Clark, a US herbalist, has also benefited from MetaPhase. Though not a diagnosed diabetic, he has experienced firsthand the battle between insulin resistance and trying to keep his weight down. He lost 8 pounds after just 15 days of taking MetaPhase at the maximum dosage. The only 'side effect' was a noticeable spike in energy, without the jitters attributable to your typical diet formula. But that's because MetaPhase isn't a diet formula.

When your body is balanced and functioning properly, it produces enough insulin to move blood sugar into your cells to be used as energy. When your bloodstream is continually saturated with an excess of sugar, however, your cells will begin to adapt, becoming less and less responsive to the insulin.

As a result, sugar remains in the bloodstream – prompting your pancreas to produce even more insulin in an effort to clear it out. Meanwhile, the hypothalamus, another organ essential to the body's lifelong balancing act, senses the presence of these unusually large amounts of insulin.

The hypothalamus sends out signals for more sugar to eliminate the excess insulin – all in the form of a hunger pang. In particular it produces cravings for sugary foods like chocolate, biscuits and bagels. The fix is a fast but inefficient one. Blood sugar levels continue to soar, but without the metabolic support to process glucose efficiently, the body is chronically devoid of the energy that it needs to function.

MetaPhase assists in the repair of the very system that regulates insulin and glucose levels within the body, while keeping your mood calm and collected. And it curbs the uncontrollable sugar and carbohydrate cravings that do nothing but add fuel to the fire.

Restoring balance, preserving health

If that were the extent of it, MetaPhase would still be an invaluable addition to the anti-diabetes arsenal. But it's got one more trick up its sleeve.

MetaPhase also offers support for type 1 diabetics whose pancreases don't produce any insulin at all. Although there is no cure for this particular condition, tight control of glucose levels in the blood limits the damage caused by excess sugar, and, in turn, inhibits the numerous complications associated with the disease.

Patton Whittington, a type 1 diabetic with volatile blood sugar levels subject to drastic peaks and valleys, decided to take MetaPhase. In the past, he'd tried a variety of so-called 'kitchen sink' remedies in conjunction with his daily insulin injections, but to little or no effect. MetaPhase, however, proved to be an exception.

Within a week, he began to notice a lowering of his glucose readings – especially after meals, when he was at his most vulnerable. In fact, its effects were so powerful that he was forced to eliminate his evening dosage, due to his blood sugar dropping too low overnight (a possibility that makes it absolutely crucial to work closely with your doctor if you decide to try MetaPhase). And his 7-pound weight loss since starting the treatment has been an added bonus.

What to take for best results

The recommended dosage for MetaPhase is one to three capsules taken 20 minutes before meals, three times a day. Typically, you will start noticing results within three to four weeks, although it may take up to eight weeks. After three to five months of regular use, a maintenance dosage of one capsule twice a day before your morning and afternoon meal will help regulate your glucose metabolism.

As already mentioned, it is extremely important that you work closely with your doctor if you decide to use MetaPhase, as the dosage of your type 1 or type 2 medication may need to be altered as your blood sugar levels drop.

- **Discover how the leaves of the banaba tree can help regulate blood sugar levels and encourage weight-loss**

GlucoFit (formerly known as GlucoTrim and Glucosol), a herbal extract of the leaves of the banaba tree, can help manage diabetes. Traditional uses of the banaba tree, which grows in India, Southeast Asia and the Philippines, include brewing tea from the leaves as a treatment for diabetes and hyperglycaemia (elevated blood sugar).

Today, supplementation with GlucoFit has been clinically proven to help type 2 diabetes sufferers by aiding blood sugar maintenance. In addition, studies indicate that it may promote weight-loss too.

GlucoFit is unique in encouraging glucose uptake in your cells

Corosolic acid is the active plant chemical present in GlucoFit. It has been found to regulate blood sugar by improving glucose metabolism and activating glucose transport into cells.

Your cell membranes contain various glucose 'transporters' or carrier molecules that regulate the level of glucose within your cells. Insulin, the main hormone associated with blood sugar balance, increases glucose-transporter activity, promoting the uptake of sugar from your blood. When insulin production is impaired, as in the case of diabetes, glucose is not taken up by the cells from your blood as it should be, resulting in raised blood sugar.

GlucoFit is considered to have an insulin-like action because, like insulin, it promotes the uptake of glucose from the blood into the cells. Unlike insulin (which must be injected), GlucoFit can be taken orally because it is not broken down in the gut.

To date, very few compounds have been known to affect glucose transport activity, which is why scientists are so excited about GlucoFit. It regulates blood sugar levels and promotes normal blood sugar without causing hypoglycaemia.

Taking 48mg of soft gel GlucoFit tablets has been found most effective

A randomised, double-blind crossover study with 12 type 2 diabetic patients taking 48mg of GlucoFit a day, was found to promote normal blood glucose metabolism ((*Biosci Biotechnol Biochem. 1996;60:204-208; Southeastern Institute of BioMedical Research, Inc. Bradenton, FL, Study 08-99, Glucosol Blood Glucose Study in Normal volunteers, submitted, November 29, 1999*). It also showed that GlucoFit's benefits were sustained for several weeks even after discontinuation of the supplement.

In addition, a series of clinical studies, conducted in 1999 by Dr. William Judy at the Southeastern Institute of Biomedical Research in Florida, showed significant benefits of GlucoFit supplementation in diabetic patients.

In a three-part study involving 10 type 2 diabetic patients, the higher the daily dose of GlucoFit, the greater the fall in blood glucose levels (*Biosci Biotechnol Biochem. 1996;60:204-208; Southeastern Institute of BioMedical Research, Inc. Bradenton, FL, Study 08-99, Glucosol Blood Glucose Study in Normal volunteers, submitted, November 29, 1999).* The subjects were divided into two groups of five. In the first part of the study they were given 16mg of GlucoFit daily for two weeks, then 32mg a day, and finally 48mg a day. There was a two week wash-out period between each increase in dosage.

One group was given GlucoFit in the form of an oil-based soft gel and the other group was given the product in the form of a dry powder in a hard gelatine capsule.

The findings showed that not only was there a greater decrease in blood sugar at the higher dosage – 31.9 per cent drop with 48mg compared to 3.18 per cent with 16mg and 6.5 per cent with 32mg – but GlucoFit was more effective when provided in an oil-based soft gel, rather than a dry powder formulation.

Low-calorie diet plus GlucoFit resulted in 4.8lbs weight loss in only 30 days!

In addition to normalising blood sugar levels, the type 2 trial participants (taking the soft gel formulation) experienced an average weight loss of 3.2 pounds. This effect is believed to be associated with the release of the hormone glucagon by the pancreas, which stimulates the breakdown of fat into free fatty acids. These fatty acids are converted into glycerol and then into glucose which is released into the blood. GlucoFit may contribute to the efficient transport of these blood sugars into cells for conversion to energy.

Type 2 diabetic patients on a restricted calorie intake diet and exercise regime were able to lose more weight while taking GlucoFit. The average weight loss was 4.8 pounds in 30 days.

As in the case of diabetic patients, it was noted that GlucoFit seems to induce weight loss in non-diabetic individuals as well. After a 15- and 30-day course of GlucoFit, the average weight loss was 1.25 pounds and 2.4 pounds respectively. Interestingly, two weeks after GlucoFit supplementation had stopped, an average weight loss of 2.6 pounds was measured. Blood sugar levels in non-diabetics were also found to remain in the normal range both before and after a 30-day course of GlucoFit (48mg per day). These findings confirm that GlucoFit is safe to take and does not lower blood sugar levels in healthy individuals.

What to take for best results

The suggested dose is one softgel (each capsule contains 0.24mg of corosolic acid) half an hour before morning and evening meals, or as otherwise directed by a healthcare practitioner. Diabetics who manage their disease through diet, and those who rely on insulin or other conventional diabetic drugs, must consult their GP before using GlucoFit, as it may alter the dose of medication required.

• **Protect yourself against the common culprit scientists believe is behind a range of serious diseases from diabetes to Alzheimer's**

In the last decade, scientists have realised that a common factor lies behind a host of chronic illnesses that doctors typically treat in isolation: Inflammation. To most of us, inflammation is what happens when we get a mosquito bite, or a wound becomes infected, or we hit our thumb with a hammer. Your immune system kicks into action, white blood cells rush to the site and there is swelling, pain and a feeling of heat.

This same process is now thought to play a key role in illnesses as diverse as osteoarthritis, heart disease, irritable bowel syndrome, multiple sclerosis, Alzheimer's disease, depression, certain types of cancer... and, as mentioned on page 13, diabetes.

Chronic inflammation is insidious and often invisible. You don't feel any pain or fever and you may not think you are ill, but it is like a fire quietly smouldering within you, upsetting the delicate balance between your major body systems: endocrine, nervous, digestive, cardiovascular and respiratory.

In a healthy body, these systems constantly communicate with each other, but with chronic inflammation that communication becomes distorted and disease is the end result.

Inflammation becomes chronic in response to a persistent stimulus, such as a low-grade, lingering infection, a food allergy, the constant assault of free radicals from a junk food diet, or a growing body burden of heavy metals, pesticides, and other chemicals. It could even be ongoing psychological stress or insufficient sleep.

One of the adverse effects of chronic inflammation is the destruction of the insulin-producing beta-cells in the pancreas, which causes type 1 diabetes when it involves an auto-immune condition, and type 2 diabetes when it results from a metabolic imbalance.

Cherry Turmeric Complex was developed in response to the growing problem of chronic inflammation. It contains a combination of botanical compounds – including extracts of Montmorency cherries, turmeric root, ginger root and black pepper, together with cayenne powder and quercetin – that have all been extensively researched for their anti-inflammatory properties.

Plant compounds block inflammation in the same way as COX-2 inhibitor drugs... but without the side effects

Non-steroidal anti-inflammatory drugs (NSAIDs) are the standard treatment for inflammatory problems. They block the action of an enzyme called cyclo-oxygenase (COX), which is involved in the production of chemicals called prostaglandins, some of which cause pain and inflammation in the body. Common NSAIDs are aspirin, ibuprofen and diclofenac.

The downside is that NSAIDs block two variants of the COX enzyme, called COX-1 and COX-2. Blocking COX-1 has the side effect of stomach irritation and bleeding, which can lead to a peptic ulcer. To overcome this, COX-2 inhibitor drugs were developed, which target only that variant of the enzyme. Celecoxib (Celebrex) is a COX-2 inhibitor commonly used to relieve the pain and inflammation of osteoarthritis and rheumatoid arthritis. However, even COX-2 drugs have unpleasant side effects, including abdominal pain, diarrhoea, flatulence, nausea, dizziness and insomnia.

Several of the natural compounds in Cherry Turmeric Complex act in exactly the same way as COX-2 drugs to block inflammation, but without the unwanted side effects. Unlike pharmaceutical drugs, the ingredients in the formula provide nutrients and antioxidants that promote overall good health:

Montmorency sour cherries are rich in polyphenolic antioxidant compounds, such as anthocyanins, which help fight the free radicals that cause oxidative damage to our cells (*Crit Rev Food Sci Nutr. 2011 Jan; 51 (1): 1-12*). Anthocyanins block the COX enzymes that produce inflammatory prostaglandins in a manner comparable to ibuprofen (*Phytomedicine. 2001 Sep; 8 (5): 362-9*). Montmorency cherries also contain a flavonoid called cyanidin, which has been shown to have better anti-inflammatory activity than aspirin, while protecting the stomach lining from damage (*Phytochem Anal. 2005 May-Jun; 16(3): 175-80*).

Curcumin is the active ingredient of turmeric root, a bright yellow curry spice, and is a potent anti-inflammatory compound. It has been the subject of intensive research in recent years for its anti-cancer properties. In numerous studies, curcumin has been shown to inhibit NF kappa-B, a major cellular inflammatory agent (*J Biol Chem. 2011 Jun 14. [Epub ahead of print]*).

Research also shows that curcumin strongly suppresses the COX-2 enzyme, so reducing inflammation, without the side-effects of popular COX-2 inhibitor drugs (*J Physiol Pharmacol. 2011 Feb; 62 (1): 21-8*). Evidence from clinical trials supports the use of curcumin for people with rheumatoid arthritis, psoriasis and inflammatory bowel disease (*J Fam Pract. 2011 Mar; 60 (3): 155-6*).

Black pepper contains an alkaloid called piperine, which has been found to inhibit the development of cancer cells, alleviate high blood pressure, regulate bowel movements and to have antidepressant-like effects in animal studies. It has been added to the formula for its ability to switch on receptors in the brain (called TRPV1 receptors) that control how nutrients are absorbed and distributed in the body. Specifically, research has shown that curcumin becomes an incredible 20 times more bioavailable when taken together with piperine (*Planta Med. 1998 May; 64 (4): 353-6*).

Capsaicin (responsible for the spicy heat of cayenne pepper), like piperine, affects the TRPV1 receptor system, but in a different way. In 1997, a research team at the University of California showed that capsaicin selectively attaches itself to the TRPV1 protein and activates heat sensitive neurons in the nervous system (*Nature 1997 Oct; 389: 816–24*). Prolonged activation of these neurons desensitises them so that pain from inflammation in the body is reduced. Capsaicin has been used to reduce the pain of inflammatory conditions including arthritis, psoriasis and irritable bowel syndrome.

Ginger, like turmeric, is a root used in Indian cooking that has demonstrated anti-inflammatory properties in several studies. The active ingredients are compounds called gingerols and shogaols, which recent research at the University of Illinois in Chicago has shown to be COX-2 inhibitors (*Fitoterapia. 2011 Jan; 82 (1): 38-43*). In addition, the compound zingerone in ginger root acts as an antioxidant and, like curcumin, has been shown to inhibit NF kappa-B (*Exp Gerontol. 2010 Jun; 45 (6): 419-26*). It can also reduce arthritis pain... when 250 people with knee osteoarthritis were given a standardized ginger extract or placebo over a six week period, an impressive two-thirds of those taking the ginger extract reported relief from pain (*Arthritis Rheum. 2001 Nov; 44 (11): 2531-8*).

Quercetin is a natural plant flavonoid, recognised for its ability to reduce levels of inflammatory leukotrienes and histamine (*Inflamm Allergy Drug Targets. 2010 Sep; 9 (4): 263-85*). New research from the Netherlands has shown that quercetin could reduce heart disease risk by lowering levels of C-reactive protein and other inflammatory compounds, as well as reducing plaque build-up in the arteries (*Atherosclerosis. 2011 May 5. [Epub ahead of print]*).

What to take for best results

The recommended dose is one Cherry Turmeric Complex vegicap daily, with food. If you are pregnant, breastfeeding or taking prescription medication, you should talk to your doctor before taking this supplement.

- **Reformulated blood sugar-lowering supplement is 300% more effective just by adding one new ingredient, cinnamon**

Back in 2002, world-renowned formulator, Jon Barron's goal was to help people lower their blood sugar. So he formulated a product called Glucotor, designed to help people with sugar management problems such as diabetes. At that time, he considered including cinnamon in his formula.

But at the time Barron was working on Glucotor, cinnamon wasn't practical for most people as a sugar management supplement, as you would need anywhere from half to one heaped teaspoon a day to get the desired effect, and as small as that amount seems, adding that much to the existing formula would mean taking as many as 18 capsules a day. Also, when you start taking cinnamon at those levels, it has potential side-effects of bronchial constriction, skin rashes, and inflammation.

So Barron's original Glucotor formula went cinnamon-less. Since then, Glucotor has racked up an 82 per cent success rate... a result most people would be satisfied with. But Barron wasn't. So he decided to reformulate Glucotor. The result is a product called Glucotor-2, which includes an all-natural ingredient that has been proven to boost the body's insulin response 20-fold. This one addition to the original formula has made the already impressive Glucotor up to 300 per cent more effective than similar products without the potential of toxic side-effects.

Make your insulin receptors more receptive

But why reformulate at all when you've already got something with such a high success rate? Simply put, Barron says the success rate just wasn't high enough considering it's a human statistic. He couldn't see past the 18 per cent of people that he wasn't helping.

That led him on a search for other ingredients he could add to boost Glucotor's effectiveness. And once again, he arrived back at cinnamon. But this time he found a specific cinnamon extract, called Cinnulin PF, which eliminated the roadblocks he'd encountered before.

In diabetes, either the body doesn't produce enough insulin or the cells resist it, so the sugar remains in the blood, builds up to higher and higher levels, and ultimately starts damaging protein-based tissue and organs. Cinnulin PF helps trigger receptor sensitivity to insulin and prime the receptor for glucose uptake.

So just what is Cinnulin PF? Well, as Barron puts it: "It's pretty amazing. It's a patented cinnamon extract that operates at the cellular and molecular levels. It actually works to make the insulin receptor sites on your individual body cells more receptive. If you have enough cinnamon every day, you can actually increase your body's insulin response three-fold. That's 300 per cent – and that's a big deal."

All the benefit, none of the risks

Until recently methyl-hydroxy-chalcone polymer (or MHCP) was thought to be the active compound in cinnamon responsible for the beneficial effect on blood glucose. It turns out that early research misidentified the substances responsible for these actions as cinnamon's MHCP fractions. The substances actually providing the blood sugar-lowering benefits are water-soluble polyphenol polymers called Type-A polymers (*J Agric Food Chem 2004; 52 (1): 65-70*).

Integrity Nutraceuticals International (INI), a raw material supplier of bulk nutraceuticals and specialty compounds like Cinnulin PF, created a water-based cinnamon extract using a process that removes the potentially harmful compounds from whole cinnamon while leaving the Type-A polymers intact. This process doesn't use chemical solvents. Extracts made with solvents other than water contain photochemicals that are more likely to be toxic at higher doses.

This process makes Cinnulin PF stronger: The lipid soluble portion of cinnamon has been shown to have no effect on glucose metabolism. But in contrast, the water-soluble portion has been proven to increase glucose uptake by 20-fold.

Early research looks promising, a 29% reduction in fasting glucose levels

In one study, researchers tested cinnamon's effects by using a water-based cinnamon extract similar to Cinnulin PF on 28 people with type 2 diabetes.

Patients received 500 milligrams of a formula containing water extracts of cinnamon, heshouwu, and mushroom three times per day. Another 29 patients were given a placebo. After two months, researchers found that subjects in the treatment group had a 15 per cent reduction in fasting glucose (a measurement of the blood glucose in the morning prior to the ingestion of any food for the previous 12 hours) (*FASEB J 2002; 16 (4) : A647*).

In another study, 60 type 2 diabetics were divided into six groups: three placebo groups and three experimental groups. Participants took 1, 3, or 6 grams of cinnamon daily or the placebo. After 40 days, participants in the cinnamon groups had 18 to 29 per cent drops in their fasting glucose. They also experienced 20 to 30 per cent lower triglycerides, 7 to 27 per cent reductions in LDL cholesterol, and 12 to 26 per cent lower total cholesterol levels (*Diabetes Care 2003; 26 (12): 3, 215-18*). There were no significant changes in any of the placebo groups.

However, all of the patients in the study were also taking oral hypoglycaemic (blood sugar-lowering) medications, so it's hard to say for sure in this case if cinnamon was the sole factor in the improvements.

What to take for best results

Glucotor-2 can be taken by people with either type 1 or type 2 diabetes. The recommended dosage for Glucotor-2 with Cinnulin PF is one or two capsules five to 10 minutes before eating. If you're currently taking medications for blood sugar, cholesterol, or heart disease, talk to your doctor before trying this formula. Barron did note that some people have a problem digesting the capsules quickly enough to get the blood sugar-lowering effects. The problem, as Barron explains, is that many people, particularly as they get older, have burned out their ability to produce stomach acid. Once you get to that point, you no longer have enough stomach acid to easily break down capsules: It takes so long that the Glucotor can't get in place soon enough to block the receptor sites. But taking the formula out of the capsules lets you bypass that problem. So, if you don't get the results you expect, try taking the Glucotor-2 powder out of the capsules and mixing it with a little apple sauce or a small glass of water.

• **Meet PteroMax... the newcomer that could cut your risk of diabetes, heart disease and cancer and improve your brain function, too**

Scientists believe that an exciting new, natural compound could help significantly reduce your chances of developing diabetes, cancer and cardiovascular disease, in addition to lowering inflammation and improving brain function. Its name is pterostilbene and it is now available in the UK as PteroMax, a supplement produced by leading 'bioceutical' manufacturer Biotivia.

Pterostilbene is an astonishing compound that has been identified as the molecule in blueberries responsible for their health benefits. Like its close chemical relative resveratrol, the heart-protecting ingredient in red grape skins, it belongs to a group of compounds called stilbenes.

PteroMax combines the power of both pterostilbene and resveratrol with another stilbene called polydatin and a complex of polyphenols from red wine grapes, green tea and Japanese knotweed. Polyphenols are potent antioxidants that protect the body from damaging free radicals. PteroMax is the world's first high-strength multi-stilbene and multi-polyphenol supplement and its synergistic formulation promises health benefits that go far beyond those of resveratrol alone.

Incredibly, just one capsule of PteroMax contains more pterostilbene than 100kg (220 pounds) of organic blueberries, as well as more resveratrol than is contained in a dozen bottles of red wine, more polydatin than 500kg (1,100 pounds) of grapes, and a full spectrum of natural polyphenols.

Although the research on pterostilbene has so far been confined to laboratory experiments and animal trials, scientists worldwide are eagerly investigating pterostilbene's potential to combat a wide range of major diseases. Chemist, Agnes Rimando, of the US Agricultural Research Service, says: "The more we study pterostilbene, the more we see its huge potential in the human health field". One area where it is showing enormous promise is as a natural anti-cancer agent (*J Agric Food Chem. 2011 Mar 23; 59 (6): 2725-33*).

Pterostilbene helps lower blood sugar and cholesterol levels

Improving blood sugar control and preventing diabetes could be another health benefit of pterostilbene. When scientists fed normal and diabetic rats a diet supplemented with pterostilbene, it significantly reduced blood glucose and increased insulin levels (*Life Sci. 2006 Jul 10; 79(7): 641-5*). It also reduced levels of specific liver enzymes used to indicate insulin resistance and diabetes.

Pterostilbene is also showing promise in the fight against a diabetes-related complication, heart and circulatory disease. When it was added to the diet of hamsters with high cholesterol levels, their LDL ('bad') cholesterol dropped by 29 per cent, while HDL ('good') cholesterol went up seven per cent, compared with a control group (*J Agric Food Chem. 2005 May 4; 53 (9): 3403-7*).

The compound may further help circulatory health by preventing the changes to artery walls that lead to atherosclerosis (hardening of the arteries) and high blood pressure. In animal studies, it inhibited the artificially-induced abnormal growth of arterial cells by suppressing the action of an enzyme called Akt kinase (*Vascul Pharmacol. 2010 Jul-Aug; 53(1-2): 61-7*).

Another trick pterostilbene appears to have up its sleeve is the ability to reduce the effects of ageing and reverse age-related memory and coordination problems. After being fed pterostilbene for eight weeks, elderly rats (equivalent to 70-75 years old in human terms) performed significantly better in motor function and memory tests (*J Agric Food Chem. 2008 Nov 26; 56 (22): 10544-51*).

Although pterostilbene is the star player in PteroMax, a new study from Italy has shown that both resveratrol and polydatin are able to powerfully suppress the inflammatory processes that lie at the root of many chronic diseases (*Inflammation. 2011 Mar 3. [Epub ahead of print]*).

What to take for best results

The recommended dose of PteroMax is one capsule a day, taken each morning on waking, at least 45 minutes prior to having breakfast. Although the ingredients in PteroMax are safe, even at extremely high doses, it is not recommended for use by children under 12 or by pregnant or lactating women, without the advice of a doctor.

- **How news of a 'super food' from Japan is quickly spreading... make sure you don't miss out on its many benefits**

You've probably read or heard the phrase "Let food be thy medicine". Uttered by Hippocrates, the 'Father of Medicine', more than two thousand years ago, today his famous words now hold more truth and credibility than ever before. This follows extensive scientific research that is continually uncovering incredible health-related benefits linked to a wide range of foods from all over the globe.

One food in particular that has been found to possess many medicinal properties, despite remaining relatively unheard of in the West, is Ashitaba (*Angelica Keiskei Koidzmi*).

Indigenous to China and the Japanese islands of Izu, Ashitaba has been an important part of the local diet for hundreds of years – used as a vegetable accompaniment at meal times and also drunk as a tea.

Ashitaba is a celery-like plant belonging to the Angelica family. Because it grows very fast, in the Japanese language it literally means 'leaves of tomorrow'. Now, mounting evidence suggests it may well prove to be an essential healing agent of tomorrow and indeed in the longer-term too.

Available in supplement form, Ashitaba can help improve your overall health as well as help treat a number of medical complaints. These include type 1 and type 2 diabetes, weakened immunity, bacterial or viral infections, high blood pressure, high cholesterol, and joint or muscular pain. It also promotes detoxification of the blood, liver and kidneys.

Why Ashitaba is an ideal food for vegans and vegetarians

It is not difficult to ascertain why Ashitaba exerts so many positive effects on health when you consider the broad range of nutrients it contains –

including 11 different types of vitamins and 13 minerals.

Nutritional analysis reveals that 100 grams of Ashitaba powder contains the beta-carotene content equivalent to four carrots, the vitamin B2 content equivalent to 28 cloves of garlic, the vitamin C content equivalent to 4 lemons, and nine times the amount of iron found in spinach. It also contains vitamins B1, B3, B5, B6, biotin, folic acid, and the minerals calcium, magnesium, potassium, phosphorous, zinc, copper, manganese, sulphur and silicon.

Most plants are devoid of vitamin B12, which is normally only obtainable through meat, fish and eggs. However, Ashitaba is a good source of this nutrient, making it an ideal supplement for strict vegetarians and vegans, who omit these foods from their diets and are at risk of suffering from a deficiency. A shortage of B12 can cause serious cognitive and nervous system problems, in addition to increasing the risk of cardiovascular disease and pernicious anaemia.

The list of therapeutic compounds in Ashitaba is endless

Many researchers believe that Ashitaba is effective against so many different medical problems as a result of its synergistic action – a combined effect of its various active components working together. In addition to the vitamins and minerals it contains, Ashitaba also possesses lesser-known nutrients that also have specific health-related benefits. These include:

- **Chlorophyll.** Ashitaba is rich in chlorophyll, the green pigment present in plants that is responsible for collecting and storing energy from the sun. Because the chlorophyll molecule is almost identical to the haemoglobin molecule in red blood cells it is often referred to as 'nature's blood'. And one of its many attributes includes its ability to stimulate the production of red blood cells, which carry oxygen to the body's tissues. It is also an excellent agent for cleansing the blood and liver, and promotes the growth of 'friendly' intestinal bacteria.

- **Germanium**. This trace mineral has been found to promote the production of interferon, a substance produced in the body that works to prevent viruses and bacteria from penetrating the body's cells.

- **Coumarins.** These are potent antioxidants, which have been found to contain anti-carcinogenic properties (*Carcinogenesis 1997; 18: 1521-1527*). They are particularly abundant in Ashitaba and other foods such as citrus fruit and celery.

- **Chalcones.** Unique to Ashitaba is a class of flavonoid compounds called chalcones. Research has shown that they are potent antioxidants, protecting cells from free radical damage, which is associated with accelerating the ageing process and with many degenerative diseases, including cancer (*Okuyama T, Takata M, Takayasu J et al. Anti-tumour-promotion by principles obtained from Angelica Keiskei. Department of Pharmacognosy and Phytochemistry, Meiji College and Pharmacy, Tokyo, Japan*). They also suppress the excessive secretion of gastric juice in the stomach, which is often caused by stress and can lead to stomach ulcers. In addition they help strengthen the immune system, regulate blood pressure and cholesterol, and exhibit anti-viral and anti-bacterial activities (*Murakami S, Kijima H, Isobe Y, Muramatsu M, Aihara H, Otomo S, Baba K, Kozawa M ; Inamori Y, Baba K, Tsujibo H, et al. Antibacterial activity of two chalcones, xanthoangelol and 4-hydroxyderricin, isolated from the root of Angelica Keiskei Koidzumi. Osaka University of Pharmaceutical Sciences, Japan*).
Chalcones have also been found to stimulate the production of Nerve Growth Factor (NGF), which is synthesised in minute amounts in the body and is essential in the development and survival of certain neurons (nerve cells) in the peripheral and central nervous system. NGF is believed to have the potential to alleviate Alzheimer's disease and peripheral neuropathy (a common neurological disorder resulting from damage to the peripheral nerves, which originate from the brain and spinal cord). In an animal study conducted by the Biomedical Group, in Takara, Japan, there was a 20 per cent increase in NGF concentration after taking Ashitaba for just four days (*www.nytimes.*

com/2001/01/15/health/AP-Brain-Exercises.html).

Helps disarm harmful free radicals and keeps blood sugar levels stable

Research published in the September 2002 issue of *Nutraceuticals World*, showed that Ashitaba out-performed a range of herbs including sage, St. John's wort, camomile, dandelion, fennel, black tea and green tea for its antioxidant potential.

There is also mounting data to suggest that Ashitaba has a regulating effect on blood sugar levels. In reviewing Ashibata, Dr. Kevin Lance Jones, a licensed acupuncturist and orthomolecular medical doctor (OMD) from California, in the US, says: "There is a patient in Texas that has insulin-dependent (type 1) diabetes that is currently taking the herb. He says that he now has to use less insulin because his blood sugar no longer spikes with attacks of hyperglycaemia. Another diabetes patient in Japan took Ashitaba for six months and his blood sugar level dropped from 400 mg/dl to 150 mg/dl."

What to take for best results

The recommended dosage is one teaspoon of Ashitaba powder taken in the morning and evening in a small amount of juice, followed by a glass of water. Ashitaba has a sweet herb-like taste and has no known contraindications. However, as with all remedies you should consult your doctor before taking Ashitaba if you are currently on any medication.

- ## Serranol launches a four-pronged attack against a range of age-related diseases... from diabetes and cancer to arthritis and Alzheimer's

As we get older the threat of age-related conditions such as diabetes, high blood pressure, heart disease, arthritis, lowered immunity, cancer and Alzheimer's disease becomes far more real.

Imagine if just one 'super supplement' could deal with all these potential threats and give you more energy, too? Now, there's a breakthrough new formula which fights premature ageing and poor health in a unique combination of ways, whilst replenishing lowered immunity and energy levels.

Serranol is packed with four of the most powerful natural ingredients available – combining the amazing, health-giving properties of Ecklonia cava extract with serrapeptase, curcumin, and vitamin D.

The research findings on Ecklonia cava speak for themselves...

The new star performer in Serranol is an edible seaweed called Ecklonia cava, also known as 'Seanol'. It's been the focus of numerous studies in recent years, which have revealed its incredible health benefits across a wide spectrum of disease conditions.

In animal experiments, Seanol has been found to be anti-diabetic, by preventing blood sugar from rising too high after meals and by protecting cells from the oxidative damage caused by high blood sugar levels (*Food Chem Toxicol. 2010 Oct; 48 (10): 2633-7; Toxicol In Vitro. 2010 Mar; 24 (2): 375-81*).

In addition, Seanol acts in exactly the same way as ACE (angiotensin-converting enzyme) inhibitor drugs in lowering blood pressure, a major risk factor for heart disease (*Nutr Res Pract. 2011 Apr; 5 (2): 93-100*).

Scientists have also discovered Seanol's ability to support the immune system by activating lymphocytes, the immune cells that detect and destroy invading pathogens (*Mar Biotechnol (NY). 2011 Feb; 13 (1): 66-73*). In addition, it is antibacterial against deadly MRSA and Salmonella strains and antiviral against the HIV-1 virus (*Foodborne Pathog Dis. 2010 Apr; 7(4): 435-41; Bioorg Med Chem. 2008 Sep 1; 16 (17): 7921-6*). If that weren't enough, Seanol has also been found to inhibit the growth of human breast cancer cells (*Food Chem Toxicol. 2009 Jul; 47 (7): 1653-8*).

The list of Seanol's potential health benefits just goes on and on, including the relief of pain and inflammation (*J Agric Food Chem. 2009 May 27; 57 (10): 4439-46*), reduction of osteoarthritis symptoms (*Arch Pharm Res. 2006 Feb; 29 (2): 165-71*), suppression of allergic reactions (*Food Chem Toxicol. 2009 Mar; 47 (3): 555-60*) and relief of asthma (*Biomed Pharmacother. 2008 Jun; 62 (5): 289-96*). Trials with college students in South Korea found that Seanol significantly improved their energy and endurance during intense physical exercise (*Int J Sport Nutr Exerc Metab. 2010 Feb; 20 (1): 72-9*).

It is important to note that two kinds of Seanol are manufactured for use in supplements and functional foods, a 13 per cent extract and a 100 per cent extract. Serranol is the only supplement available that uses the full-strength 100 per cent extract – others rely on the cheaper, but less potent, 13 per cent version.

Miracle enzyme targets the inflammation underlying many chronic diseases

Serrapeptase is a protein-digesting enzyme, which is originally isolated from silkworms – they produce it to break down their hard cocoon walls.

In the human body, serrapeptase targets dangerous protein buildups such as blood clots and arterial plaque, which can lead to a heart attack or stroke. It may also break down the amyloid-beta protein plaques in the brain that are associated with Alzheimer's disease (*Neuron. 2010; 66 (5): 695-709*). In addition, it makes the dense mucus produced in conditions like sinusitis and bronchitis less sticky, so that it is easier to expel *(Respirology. 2003 Sep; 8 (3): 316-20)*.

In the last few years, inflammation has been identified as a root cause of many chronic diseases, particularly those normally associated with ageing, such as diabetes and atherosclerosis (*Nutr Rev. 2007 Dec; 65 (12 Pt 2): S140-6*). A striking property of serrapeptase is its profound anti-inflammatory action, as shown by a clinical trial in Jordan in which serrapeptase reduced pain and swelling following the removal of wisdom teeth *(Int J Oral Maxillofac Surg. 2008 Mar; 37 (3): 264-8)*.

In other research, serrapeptase has been found to reduce inflammation and break down blood clots in a variety of ear, nose and throat disorders and to relieve the pain of carpal tunnel syndrome in 65 per cent of patients *(J Int Med Res.1990 Sep-Oct; 18 (5): 379-88; J Assoc Physicians India. 1999 Dec; 47 (12): 1170-2)*.

Curcumin and vitamin D3 help protect against diabetes, dementia and cancer

Serranol also contains a special form of bioavailable curcumin called BCM-95, which research has shown to be a massive seven times better absorbed by the human body than normal curcumin (the active principle in the Indian curry spice turmeric) *(Indian J Pharm Sci. 2008 Jul-Aug; 70(4): 445-9)*.

Scientific researchers around the world are investigating curcumin's incredible ability to fight everything from diabetes, cancer and arthritis, to cardiovascular disease, cystic fibrosis, osteoporosis and Alzheimer's disease... among many other conditions.

Studies have shown curcumin's cancer-fighting properties to be so impressive that it has been described by scientists as "one of the most powerful chemopreventive and anticancer agents". According to a recent research review, there is sufficient evidence for full scale clinical trials of curcumin in the treatment of multiple myeloma, pancreatic and colorectal cancer *(Arch Pharm (Weinheim). 2010 Sep; 343(9): 489-99)*. It has also shown great promise in the treatment of breast cancer and liver cancer.

Researchers in Japan recently described curcumin as having "outstanding anti-inflammatory and neuroprotective properties". Animal experiments have shown that curcumin protects the brain from damage following a stroke and may even protect against Alzheimer's disease by directly inhibiting the formation of amyloid-beta plaques *(Neurosci Lett. 2010 Nov*

19; 485 (2): 83-8).

The final key ingredient in Serranol is Vitamin D3, which has been the subject of numerous studies in recent years. Vitamin D deficiency is widespread in the UK and has been linked to the incidence of diabetes, cancer, hypertension, multiple sclerosis, rheumatoid arthritis, osteoporosis and muscle weakness, as well as its traditional deficiency disease, rickets, which is itself on the increase (*Nutr J. 2010 Dec 8; 9: 65*).

Restoring vitamin D to normal levels has been found to help reduce inflammation, normalise blood pressure and improve insulin sensitivity – all factors that help reduce heart disease risk (*J Clin Endocrinol Metab. 2001 Apr; 86 (4): 1633-7; QJM. 2002 Dec; 95 (12): 787-96; Prog Biophys Mol Biol. 2006 Sep; 92 (1): 39-48*). In addition, vitamin D3 supplementation has been found to reduce susceptibility to type 2 diabetes by slowing the loss of insulin sensitivity in people showing early signs of the disease (*Diabetes Care 2007; 30 (4): 980-986*).

Vitamin D also has an important role in maintaining a robust immune system. According to a recent review, "vitamin D insufficiency may lead to dysregulation of human immune responses and may therefore be an underlying cause of infectious disease and immune disorders" (*Hewison M. Vitamin D and innate and adaptive immunity. Vitam Horm. 2011; 86: 23-62*). Evidence is also piling up on vitamin D's role in preventing cancers, in particular colorectal cancer (*Cancer Epidemiol Biomarkers Prev. 2011 May; 20 (5): 1003-16*).

What to take for best results

The recommended dosage for Serranol is one capsule taken three times a day, either 30 minutes before or two hours after food.

Serranol has no known side effects or drug interactions, but women who are pregnant or breast feeding are advised to check with their doctor before taking it.

- **Discover how to safeguard your health from a diverse range of medical conditions... from diabetes to stroke**

If you're searching for a safe and effective natural remedy that can improve your overall health as well as offer protection against numerous ailments, then look no further. Taraxacum officinale, more commonly known as dandelion extract, is proving to be an excellent all-round remedy.

Taraxacum has been studied extensively during the past few years and has been found to possess a wide-range of beneficial actions. It's little wonder that it is effective against so many conditions when you consider the wealth of ingredients it contains, including flavonoids, vitamins A, C and D, resin, mucilage, magnesium, iron, potassium, inulin and polysaccharides (*Williams CA, Goldstone F, Greenham J. Phytochemistry 1996; 42: 121-127; Ling Y et al. Zhongguo Zhong Yao 1999; 24 (4): 225-226*).

They have a synergistic effect and account for taraxacum's multiple health benefits, such as helping to prevent serious conditions like heart disease, cancer and stroke. Its ability to regulate blood sugar levels also makes it beneficial for diabetics.

Taraxacum gets to work quickly and can lower blood sugar levels in just a matter of hours

Taraxacum is a useful remedy against diabetes due to its ability to prevent excess glucose from accumulating in the blood. A substance called inulin is responsible for this action. Inulin (not to be confused with the hormone insulin) is a type of fibre, which traps glucose molecules and prevents them from rising above certain safe limits in your bloodstream (*Akhtar MS et al. J Pak Med Assoc 1985;35:207-210*).

Dr. R Petlevski and his team from the Department of Medical Biochemistry and Haematology, University of Zagreb in Croatia, have studied the effects of taraxacum and other plant extracts on diabetic mice. They found that preparations containing it were extremely effective at reducing high glucose levels in the blood, lowering it by as much as 20 per cent.

The researchers were amazed to observe just how quickly this reduction occurred, as blood sugar levels were lowered only two hours after taraxacum was administered (*Petlevski R. et al. J Ethnopharmacol 2001; 75 (2-3): 181-184*).

Commenting on the findings, Dr. Petlevski says: "The extract significantly reduces glucose levels in mice and further studies are now planned to focus on the search for the active ingredients of the extracts".

A safer way to reduce fluid retention and swelling

Diuretics (water tablets) are regularly prescribed by doctors to treat high blood pressure and fluid retention. They work by eliminating unwanted fluids from the body. However, they have one major drawback in that they can also cause a loss of the mineral potassium from the kidneys, which can lead to abnormalities in heartbeat rhythm and muscle weakness.

The good news is that taraxacum acts as a diuretic but without interfering with potassium levels (*Racz-Kotilla E, Racz G, Solomon A. Planta Med 1974; 26: 212-217*). This is particularly useful for people who are trying to lose weight and who suffer from excessive fluid retention – including swollen ankles and swelling of the abdomen.

...Its list of health-related benefits just keeps on growing

New research is unveiling several hitherto unknown benefits linked to taraxacum. For example, researchers from the Department of Biological Sciences, University of Ulsan in Korea, have detected a protein molecule in it that acts as an anti-coagulant (*Yun SI, Cho HR, Choi HS. Biosci Biotechnol Biochem 2002; 66 (9): 1859-1864*).

The protein stops blood from clotting prematurely and offers promising potential as a preventative against blood clots, which increase the risk of stroke, heart attacks and thrombosis. This clot-busting protein is so new that it hasn't even been given a scientific name yet.

In addition, it's been revealed that taraxacum can block inflammatory chemicals, including interleukin-6 and tumour necrosis factor-alpha (TNF-a), that are implicated in contributing to cancer, arthritis and brain damage (*Kim HM, Shin HY et al. Immunopharmacol Immunotoxicol 2000; 22 (3): 519-530*).

What to take for best results

The recommended dose is 540mg of taraxacum taken one to three times a day. There are no reports of side effects or toxicity. However, you should be aware that people who are allergic to pollen are at risk of suffering an allergic reaction to taraxacum extract.

- ## Stop the snowball effect of metabolic syndrome – and gain control of your blood sugar levels for good

A brand new product called Insinase boasts a cutting-edge approach to controlling high blood sugar levels by stamping out the problem where it actually starts: at the cellular level.

The fact is that long-term over-eating and relying on processed meals and junk food has far reaching consequences beyond indigestion, stomach ache and putting on a few extra pounds.

It puts you at serious risk of metabolic syndrome (a condition characterized by symptoms such as obesity, insulin resistance and high blood pressure) and from there it is normally just a matter of time before full-blown type 2 diabetes develops.

A botanical cure for 'bad communication'

Insinase's formula consists of two botanical ingredients – reduced iso-alpha acid (RIAA) and Acacia. The first is better known as the active component of hops, the flowers that give beer its distinctively bitter flavour and pungent aroma. It is also a well-known sedative, digestive aid, anti-inflammatory, and antibiotic.

The second ingredient, Acacia, is available from a group of shrubs and trees native primarily to Australia, Africa and southern Asia. It has a wide range of health benefits, helping everything from toothaches, sore throats, and gingivitis to colitis, skin diseases, and – you guessed it – diabetes.

But while each of these ingredients has a long history in the way of herbal healing, their most important role in this particular formula is to function as what scientists call selective kinase response modulators – SKRMs, for short.

This means that Insinase acts directly on your kinases – a group of enzymes that work in every single cell in your body. Think of them as conductors, passing signals from the outside in such a way as to have a direct effect on how each cell will behave.

When communicating properly, your kinases work together to ensure that your body's performing all of its functions smoothly and harmoniously. But here's the catch: too many biscuits and slices of pizza can eventually cause a serious communication breakdown between your kinases.

Restore healthy responses – and reverse the damage that's already been done

In cases of metabolic syndrome, kinase signalling is affected primarily in your fat-storing cells (adipocytes) – which are also the cells most actively involved in glucose utilisation and insulin signalling.

Previously healthy kinase responses become compromised by a poor diet and too little exercise, and that eventually results in mayhem for just about every system in your body.

As mentioned earlier, metabolic syndrome is characterized by insulin resistance, which is strongly linked to obesity... which is also another symptom of the condition. But what may not be quite as obvious is how another factor enters into this disastrous equation: inflammation.

As it turns out, too many bags of crisps and evenings spent sitting on the couch can cause glycogen synthase kinase (GSK) to become over-activated. When this happens an inflammatory chemical called nuclear factor kappa B is triggered. The resulting inflammation starts shutting down your cells' sensitivity to insulin – a substance that's needed in order for your body to use glucose properly.

When your cells can't use sugar for energy, they turn to fat as the next best thing, frantically storing it as fuel for the future. Once your adipocytes can't hold any more fat, a signal goes out to your other organ systems telling them to start picking up the slack by storing some fat too.

And then you're really in trouble. The accumulated stress on your body – from obesity, to inflammation, to the inability to burn fuel properly – will send you head on into a diagnosis of diabetes in no time.

But the combination of botanicals in Insinase helps put a stop to this vicious cycle at its very beginning. It selectively restores the normal responses of several of the kinases behind your metabolic syndrome.

Clinically proven to lower blood sugar and blood fat levels

While developing Insinase, scientists tested over 200 natural substances for their influence on insulin responses in adipocytes before they selected the RIAA and Acacia combo as the best performer – especially in its ability to inhibit inflammation-causing nuclear factor kappa B.

They evaluated 91 patients – all with similar weights, blood pressure, waist and hip circumferences, and fasting and post-meal blood glucose levels – in a 12-week, double-blind, placebo-controlled study. Blood was drawn three times – on the first day, after eight weeks, and after 12 weeks – to assess the formula's effect on the various risk factors of metabolic syndrome.

As compared to the placebo group, participants in the RIAA/Acacia group experienced a significantly greater decrease in their homeostatic model assessment scores (a published measure of insulin resistance), and in their blood-triglyceride (TG) levels. High triglycerides (blood fats) are often the first sign of insulin resistance – and they remain high in diabetics.

Supplementation with the RIAA/Acacia blend also lowered participants' TG/HDL-cholesterol ratio – that is, their ratio of triglycerides to high-density lipoprotein (also known as 'good') cholesterol – while the placebo group experienced no changes in this area at all (*"Double-Blind, Placebo-Controlled Trial Examining the Effects of RIAA/Acacia Supplementation on Insulin Homeostasis" Robert H. Lerman, MD, PhD, Matthew L. Tripp, PhD, and Jeffery S. Bland, PhD. Functional Medical Research Center, the clinical arm of Metagenics, Inc., Gig Harbor*).

What to take for best results

For those with high blood sugar levels the recommended dosage for Insinase is three tablets a day. You should see results within eight to 12 weeks.

Contraindications: Insinase has a slight blood-thinning effect, so for this reason you shouldn't take it with anti-coagulant medication like Warfarin.

- ## Correct a blood sugar imbalance and prevent diabetes-related complications like heart disease

Maybe you've been told you have 'insulin resistance,' 'pre-diabetes,' or 'metabolic syndrome'. Or maybe you've already crossed the line into type 2 diabetes.

Whatever your doctor calls it, it means that your body is having a hard time maintaining normal blood glucose levels – and your system is giving you a warning to act now before things get worse.

It's important to heed this warning given the fact that diabetes can eventually put you at risk of developing serious complications like heart disease, kidney disease, nerve damage and vision loss.

With the early stages of type 2 diabetes and its subset of precursor conditions, your pancreas' ability to produce insulin (a hormone that regulates your blood sugar levels) isn't completely gone; it's just dysfunctional – and fortunately there are things you can do to correct it. This includes taking a new supplement called GlucoCare that is made up of a blend of Ayurvedic (ancient Indian) herbs, all of which have a long history of use when it comes to regulating blood sugar levels.

Ancient Indian secrets to controlling blood sugar levels naturally

GlucoCare combines over 25 Ayurvedic herbs – which have been traditionally used to regulate blood sugar metabolism, benefits which are now confirmed by scientific research – including:

Bitter gourd, **or bitter melon**. Scientists have isolated a hypoglycaemic peptide called polypeptide-P from the fruit, seeds, and skin of this Ayurvedic treatment for high blood sugar and found that it can lower raised blood sugar levels in animals (*J Nat Prod 1981; 44: 648-655*). One study showed that a specific variety of bitter gourd, called cerasee, cut blood sugar levels in half after just five hours (*Diabetes Res 1985; 2: 81-84*).

Researchers at Sri Venkateswara University in India reported that after 15 days of treatment with bitter gourd, "a significant reduction was observed in fasting blood glucose levels." Cholesterol and triglyceride levels also declined (*J Ethnopharmacol 1999; 67: 103-109*).

Bitter melon's benefits in this area aren't just confined to animals. In a study, glucose tolerance was improved in 73 per cent of type 2 diabetic patients given 2oz of bitter melon juice (*J Ethnopharmacol 1986; 17: 277-282*). In another study, 15 grams of the aqueous extract of bitter melon produced a 54 per cent decrease in post-prandial (occurring after eating) blood sugar in six patients (*Phytother Res 1993; 7: 285-289*).

Gymnema sylvestre is another common Ayurvedic herb present in GlucoCare that's well known for its ability to fight diabetes. Modern studies have revealed that an extract from the leaves of this plant may actually be able to help regenerate or repair beta cells which produce insulin.

In one study, 22 type 2 diabetes patients took 400mg of a gymnema sylvestre extract a day for 18 to 20 months in conjunction with conventional oral anti-hyperglycaemic drugs. The researchers reported that the patients showed "a significant reduction in blood glucose... and conventional drug dosage could be decreased." Five of the participants were able to discontinue their conventional drug therapy altogether and maintain normal blood sugar control with gymnema alone (*J Ethnopharmacol 1990; 30: 295-300*).

Pitasara also has some impressive research findings behind it. In an animal study, administration of a water-based pitasara extract effectively lowered blood glucose levels by 60 per cent after just 30 days. Another study showed that specific flavanoids in pitasara can also lower total cholesterol and triglycerides – important markers to watch considering the link between type 2 diabetes and heart disease (*J Nat Prod 1993; 56: 989-994*).

Ocimum Sanctum (which literally means 'holy basil') can lower fasting and post-prandial (after eating a meal) blood glucose levels. In a placebo-controlled human study, type 2 diabetes patients treated with holy basil extract saw their fasting blood glucose fall by almost 18 per cent from baseline levels, while the control group experienced no significant change (*Int J Clin Pharmacol Ther 1996; 34: 406-409*).

Eugenia jambolana – the seed and fruit pulp of this plant can also lower raised blood sugar levels. A recent study, involving animals with varying degrees of diabetes, showed a 12 per cent drop in fasting blood glucose levels after just one day of treatment with eugenia. After 15 days of treatment, those animals with mild diabetes had fasting blood glucose levels 41 per cent lower than they were at the start of the study (*J Ethnopharmacol 2003; 85: 201-206*).

Several published studies have shown that GlucoCare can effectively lower blood glucose, reduce dependence on prescription diabetes drugs, and prevent complications of diabetes like diabetic retinopathy – one of the leading causes of blindness (*Biol Pharm Bull 1994 Aug;17 (8): 1106-1110; J Nutr Sci Vitaminol 2001 Feb; 47 (1): 57-63; Diabetes Obes Metab 2002 Jan; 4 (1): 43-48*).

What to take for best results

The recommended dosage for GlucoCare is one tablet taken twice a day with meals. Please be aware that it can take several weeks before improvements are experienced. If you are already taking a prescription drug to lower your blood sugar, it is important that you talk to your doctor before taking GlucoCare.

- **This award-winning nutrient-packed powerhouse is your new weapon in the fight against metabolic syndrome**

Chlorella is a single-celled green algae that has been a popular nutritional supplement for several years and its health benefits have been confirmed by scientific studies. These include immune activation (*Cancer Immunol Immunother 1984; 17: 90–94*), growth promotion (*Biol Abstr 1972; 54: 9694*), and the prevention of stress-related ulcers (*Planta Med 1997; 63: 465–466*).

Ground-breaking human clinical trials have now been conducted in Japan that have demonstrated Chlorella's incredible ability to safeguard our health at the crucial level of gene expression, which could herald a real breakthrough in the fight against diabetes and cardiovascular disease.

Added to this, a patented new form of Chlorella – Sun Chlorella 'A' – is now available in the UK. In its natural form, Chlorella keeps all its nutrients locked inside an indigestible cell wall, but thanks to a unique, high-pressure pulverising system that blasts the cell wall open, Sun Chlorella 'A' releases its valuable nutrients so that they are easily absorbed by the body.

Sun Chlorella 'A' contains an astonishing quantity and variety of nutrients and is composed of 60 per cent pure plant protein. A daily dose contains all the essential amino acids plus vitamin A, vitamin B12, B6, vitamin D, folic acid, iron and fibre. In terms of iron content alone, a daily dose of Sun Chlorella 'A' is equivalent to more than half a pound of spinach (270g).

Sun Chlorella 'A' is voted most beneficial product in 2009

At the prestigious Institute for Optimum Nutrition awards ceremony in London in April 2009, Sun Chlorella 'A' received the award for 'most beneficial product'.

The Japanese clinical trial mentioned above (*J Med Food 2008; 11 (3): 395-404*) focused on a new field of research called nutrigenomics (the study of molecular relationships between nutrition and the response of genes, aiming to extrapolate how such subtle changes can affect human health).

Test subjects were divided into two groups, those having abnormally high blood sugar, cholesterol and triglyceride (blood fat) levels, together with low glucose tolerance, and a control group in which these levels were within the normal range. These symptoms, along with high blood pressure, are typical of metabolic syndrome.

Sun Chlorella 'A' lowers cholesterol, blood fat and blood sugar levels

Both groups took 20 Sun Chlorella 'A' tablets twice a day for 12 weeks. Blood tests were carried out at the start of the trial and at 4, 8, 12 and 16 weeks.

The test results showed that Chlorella was responsible for improving both fat metabolism and glucose metabolism and that it significantly reduced fasting blood glucose levels, body fat percentage, and blood cholesterol levels. Specifically, Sun Chlorella 'A' targeted the genes involved in glucose absorption, in a way that tended to lower blood sugar levels.

Although the researchers did not measure the participants' blood pressure, an earlier US study carried out at Virginia Medical College (VMC), suggests that Sun Chlorella 'A' can also help keep high blood pressure under control (*J Med Food 2002; 5 (3): 141-152*).

In the VMC study, people with mild to moderate hypertension took 50 Sun Chlorella tablets, plus 100ml of liquid Chlorella extract (Sun Chlorella Wakasa Gold), every day for two months. All other blood pressure medication was stopped from one month before the start of the trial.

Results showed that 25 per cent of the participants responded extremely well to the treatment and achieved their goal of a diastolic blood pressure reading of 90 or below. For the other 75 per cent, blood pressure improvements were only small. While the researchers could not explain this wide variation, it may have been caused by differences in people's responses to stopping their regular medication.

The VMC study also looked at cholesterol and triglyceride levels, and, like the Japanese clinical trial, found that both showed reductions, with particularly significant drops in total cholesterol and LDL cholesterol (the dangerous kind). In addition, quality of life questionnaires revealed an overall perception that health had significantly improved as a result of

Chlorella consumption.

The results of these two trials show that Sun Chlorella 'A' could offer an effective, safe and natural treatment for people who need to reduce cholesterol and blood fat levels and improve their blood sugar control.

What to take for best results

If you are not used to taking Chlorella, begin gradually by taking five of the little Sun Chlorella 'A' tablets a day for the first week, then increase to 10 a day in the second week, building up to 15 to 30 tablets daily, according to your health needs. It is advisable to split the dosage (e.g. five tablets, three times a day) to maximise the benefit. Chlorella is very safe and generally free from side effects. You should talk to your doctor before stopping or reducing any prescription medication.

• Lose fat that is putting your health at risk

Abdominal fat is the hardest fat to get rid of. Well, it was – until now. Participants in a recent 12-week trial whittled down their waistlines and shed pounds – while the control group actually gained weight.

The best part was that nobody in this study counted a single calorie or even did a single sit-up. That's because they were taking the first natural product of its kind to shrink the 'impossible-to-lose' visceral fat that builds up around your tummy. This is good news as more and more scientists believe that losing your spare tyre could actually save your life.

Even if your body weight is normal, hidden fat could kill you

As mentioned previously, metabolic syndrome is a condition in which blood lipids, blood glucose, and blood pressure are poorly controlled. It is gaining recognition as a major indicator of diseases including coronary artery disease, heart attack, diabetes, stroke and even cancer. One of the most visible indicators of metabolic syndrome is visceral fat – the fat that collects deep around the vital organs in your abdomen, resulting in an expanding waistline or 'middle age spread' (*Endocrinol. Metab Clin N Amer. 2006; 33 (2): 351-375*).

Frighteningly, even normal-weight people with increased visceral fat tend to have high blood pressure, elevated levels of insulin and blood fats and increased risk factors for inflammatory and cardiovascular disease. A study of 387 normal-weight people showed that men with waists measuring 40 inches doubled their risk of dying prematurely, and women with waists measuring 35 inches were 79 per cent more likely to die than women with 28-inch waists (*NEJM 2008; 359 (20): 2105-2120*).

What's more, studies have shown that higher blood sugar levels are associated with lower cognitive function and people with diabetes have a 1.5 times higher chance of experiencing dementia (*Psychol Ageing 2009; 24 (1): 154-162*).

Amazing liquorice root extract breaks down your spare tyre

Researchers first recognised the link between visceral fat and metabolic syndrome when, in a preliminary study, visceral fat was surgically removed from ageing rodents. The rats' insulin levels were reduced to those of young rats. There were dramatic results even with rats that were genetically predisposed to develop diabetes: removing visceral fat delayed its onset (*Gabriely I, Ma XH, Yang XM, Atzmon G, Rajala MW, Berg AH, Scherer P, Rossetti L, Barzilai N. Removal of visceral fat prevents insulin resistance and glucose intolerance of ageing: an adipokine-mediated process?*).

It appears that even modest reductions in visceral fat can help reverse the effects of metabolic syndrome. Now, a new supplement is available in the UK that could help you to shrink that spare tyre. Glabrinex, from Vitamin Research Products, is based on a flavonoid called glabridin, extracted from the root of the liquorice plant (*Glycyrrhiza glabra*), a herb with a four thousand year history of medical use.

While liquorice is known to have several beneficial health effects, it's this specific flavonoid that's been shown to reduce visceral fat. Glabridin increases the activity of enzymes that break down fat tissue. It stimulates the metabolism of fatty acids in the liver, effectively increasing your body's fat-burning ability. It also lowers the levels in blood plasma and liver tissue of fats called triglycerides, putting the brakes on the formation of visceral fat.

In addition, glabridin has an effect on cellular DNA, changing the way visceral fat cells mature. Animal studies and human clinical trials have both demonstrated that glabridin can reduce the amount of visceral fat, so helping to eliminate a major cause of metabolic syndrome.

Banish visceral fat without dieting or spending endless hours in the gym

Several studies on both animals and humans have shown glabridin's ability to reduce body weight, waist circumference and abdominal fat, to suppress the formation of visceral fat and to help control blood glucose.

In one study, obese rats fed a high-fat diet were treated with liquorice-root extract. Even on that high-fat diet, the extract significantly decreased the weight of the rats' abdominal fat tissue (*Biosci Biotechnol Biochem 2008; 72(12): 3225-3231*).

A similar study, in which diabetic mice were fed a high-fat diet, further demonstrated the extract's effect on fat. It significantly reduced body weight gain, weight of abdominal fat tissue, and blood sugar levels as compared with the control group. In yet another study on obese mice, glabridin actually shrank abdominal fat cells and improved the fatty state of liver cells.

In one human trial, researchers found that 900mg of glabridin per day resulted in very impressive drops in body weight and body mass index

(BMI) after just four weeks. These patients also lost visceral fat after eight weeks. While results were most impressive at a dosage of 900mg, the study also recorded significant reductions in fat mass when patients took just 300mg per day.

The same research team confirmed the effectiveness of glabridin at 300mg per day in a separate clinical trial, in which all the participants were moderately overweight. The group taking a placebo actually gained 2 pounds per week on average, while those taking glabridin lost weight.

Interestingly, this study was conducted in the US during the Thanksgiving and Christmas season and participants weren't required to change their eating habits or to exercise. Over the course of 12 weeks, over a quarter of the participants taking glabridin lost 2 pounds or more and their BMIs were also significantly reduced.

The researchers discovered that the change in participants' body weight in this study was specifically due to a reduction in body fat. Although glabridin showed impressive effects without any lifestyle changes, they speculate that it could be even more effective when combined with some dietary restrictions and increased physical activity.

Glabrinex is not a quick-loss crash diet pill. It's about gradually changing your body composition and finally getting rid of the deep-seated visceral fat that puts your life at risk. This might mean that you only lose five to ten per cent of your body weight, but it will do wonders for your health.

What to take for best results

The recommended dose of Glabrinex is three 100mg soft gel capsules a day, taken with your evening meal.

Flavonoids like glabridin may act as natural phytoestrogens, so consult your doctor before using this product if you are pregnant or nursing or if you are taking medication.

- **Losing weight and warding off metabolic syndrome could be as simple as putting the kettle on**

A brand new herbal tea, recently developed in Australia, can help you lose weight and, better still, prevent metabolic syndrome. A quarter of the world's adults are estimated to have metabolic syndrome, which makes them three times as likely to have a heart attack or stroke and five times as likely to develop type 2 diabetes.

Unlike many other 'so-called' slimming teas on the market today, Spearole Tea doesn't rely on herbs to produce a laxative or diuretic effect, which long-term can cause dehydration, diarrhoea and nausea. Nor does it contain ephedra – a common ingredient in many Chinese slimming teas, which can raise blood pressure and cause an irregular heartbeat.

Spearole Tea is a pleasant-tasting blend of green tea, spearmint, olive leaf and grape seed extract. According to the manufacturer, the Australian company Dr Red, one cup of Spearole Tea has the same antioxidant content as a cup of green tea plus a cup of olive leaf tea, a cup of spearmint tea and a glass of red wine!

The 4 ingredients in Spearole Tea help reduce abdominal fat and cholesterol levels

What Spearole Tea's four ingredients all have in common is the power to reduce inflammatory actions in the body, which are now recognised as a trigger for metabolic syndrome. Eating too much, physical inactivity and simply getting older all lead to the over-production of inflammatory chemicals called cytokines, which can inactivate insulin receptors on the surface of muscle cells, causing insulin resistance (*Am J Physiol Regul Integr Comp Physiol 2008; 294 (3): R673-680*). This allows blood sugar and insulin levels to rise too high, which in turn leads to the multiple factors involved in metabolic syndrome.

1. Green tea: Numerous studies have revealed that green tea, the main ingredient in Spearole Tea, can promote weight loss, lower cholesterol, and even help prevent cancer, cardiovascular disease and strokes (*Am Fam Physician 2009; 79 (7): 591-594*). What has got scientists excited recently, though, is green tea's potential to combat metabolic syndrome (*Phytochemistry 2009; 70 (1): 11-24*).

Green tea compounds called catechins, and in particular one called epigallocatechin gallate (EGCG), appear to prevent metabolic syndrome by slowing down the absorption of fat after meals and by reducing the deposit of 'visceral fat' around the organs in the abdomen (*Asia Pac J Clin Nutr 2008; 17 (Suppl) 1: 273-27*).

2. Olive leaf has potent antibacterial, antiviral and antifungal properties. Recent research confirms what farmers in Spain and Portugal already knew – that feeding olive leaves to pigs results in less fat being laid down in their meat (*Meat Science 2009; 82 (4): 438-443*). Now, researchers in Germany and Switzerland have found from human clinical studies that olive leaf extract, which contains an antioxidant polyphenol called oleuropein, can significantly reduce both blood pressure and blood cholesterol levels (*Phytotherapy Research 2008; 22 (9): 1239–1242*).

3. Grape seed extract contains a powerful mix of antioxidants, including a polyphenol called resveratrol – which is also found in much higher levels in grape skins – as well as various catechins. Only found in the grape seeds, rather than in the skins or juice, are other compounds called proanthocyanidins. In new research from the University of Tarragona in Spain, grape seed proanthocyanidins maintained normal blood fat and LDL cholesterol levels in rats fed a high-fat diet for 13 weeks, whilst levels of these markers in untreated control animals soared (*Int J Obes (Lond) 2009; 33 (9): 1007-1012*).

4. Spearmint has long been prized as a digestive aid and for its antibacterial and anti-parasitic properties. Recent research has discovered that it also has strong anti-inflammatory and antioxidant properties, and scientists in India have shown that an extract of spearmint leaves prevents chemically-induced cell mutation and protects chromosomes from damage (*Drug Chem Toxicol 2009; 32 (4): 411-416*). Such damage can cause cells to become cancerous, so spearmint may have an anti-cancer effect. Spearmint also tastes delicious and gives a cool, light flavour to Spearole Tea.

Spearole Tea could reverse the dangerous effects of a high fat, high sugar diet

When scientists at Queensland University in Brisbane, Australia, tested Spearole Tea on rats, their aim was to see whether it would have any effect in reducing blood pressure. What they found was incredible. Spearole Tea benefited not only blood pressure but every single marker for metabolic syndrome that they looked at – and not just a little bit, but right back to normal, healthy values (*Brown L. Antioxidant-enriched green tea attenuates the signs of metabolic syndrome in high carbohydrate/high fat-fed rats. 3rd World Congress on Tea and Health: Nutraceutical and Pharmaceutical Applications. December 3&4 2009, Dubai*).

The researchers added condensed milk, beef fat and fructose to the rats' normal diet for a period of 16 weeks. After eight weeks, half of the rats also got Spearole Tea in their diet. As expected, by the end of the study, the high fat, high sugar diet caused the rats in the control group to develop increased blood pressure, more abdominal fat, high blood glucose levels, increased liver enzyme production (showing liver dysfunction), fatty droplets in their livers and stiffer hearts due to collagen deposition. Their livers and hearts also showed a high degree of inflammation.

The rats that were fed Spearole Tea for the last eight weeks of the study, on the other hand, had completely normal readings from all the tests and almost no signs of inflammation in their hearts and livers. Systolic blood pressure, which was monitored throughout the study, rose steadily until week eight, after which it dropped markedly in the rats that got Spearole Tea from then on, while it continued to rise in the control group. If these results had come from the testing of a patentable drug, the pharmaceutical companies would be falling over each other to run human clinical trials and the media would be trumpeting it as a medical breakthrough!

Of course, we have to be careful when interpreting how the results of animal tests might apply to humans. Although in this case the rats developed all the symptoms of people on a high calorie, high fat diet, and the researchers cautiously suggest that overweight, mildly diabetic and mildly hypertensive patients may benefit from adding Spearole Tea to their diet. Although the rats continued to be fed an unhealthy diet throughout the trial, obviously making healthy eating choices and increasing the amount of exercise you take will only add to the beneficial effects of Spearole Tea.

What to take for best results

The recommended intake of Spearole Tea is three cups per day. Each pack contains enough tea for around 100 cups, which is over one month's supply.

- **Reverse metabolic syndrome – high blood sugar, high cholesterol and high triglycerides – with this rare Italian fruit**

A unique super citrus fruit that grows in a tiny region on the southern coast of Calabria, in Italy, possesses remarkable therapeutic properties. This small area boasts 80 per cent of the world's bergamot production – and its polyphenolic extract is exclusively used to make an antidote to metabolic syndrome.

Bergamot is different to any citrus fruit you've ever seen before. It's yellow like a lemon, but the size of an orange. It's less sour than a lemon, but much more bitter than a grapefruit.

And while you wouldn't really want to snack on bergamot, you'll probably want to consider taking it in supplement form if you suffer from metabolic syndrome.

So, what exactly makes this bitter fruit so remarkable? Well, in just 30 days, you could see astonishing study results like these:

- LDL ('bad') cholesterol level lowered by as much as 37 per cent

- 49 per cent decrease in triglycerides

- 22 per cent drop in blood sugar levels

Hard-to-control symptoms can require a nudge from Mother Nature

The fact is that, sometimes, your body needs a little help to get things right. Unfortunately, the mainstream approach often uses a battering ram where a gentle nudge would do the trick – and bergamot fruit can provide just the right nudge.

For one thing, this citrus fruit helps your body by naturally blocking one of the enzymes (HMG-CoA reductase) needed for cholesterol production. Now, your body needs cholesterol – that's why your liver makes it – but sometimes production can get a little out of control. The powerful flavonoid compounds in bergamot help keep that in check by inhibiting the HMG-CoA reductase enzyme (which gets more active when blood sugar levels are high).

Those flavonoids also impact high blood sugar levels in a very positive way. By acting directly on glucose transporter proteins and glucose-regulating enzymes, these compounds can help rein in high blood sugar as well as improving insulin sensitivity – a key factor in healthy glucose levels.

In addition, these plentiful flavonoids have well-documented antioxidant properties that contribute to your overall good health.

Bergamot is chock full of powerful, natural healing compounds

Like virtually everything produced by Mother Nature, bergamot fruit contains a wide range of healthy compounds, the most potent of which include: naringin, rutin, narirutin, hesperidin, neoeriocitrin, eriocitrin and neoesperidin.

Some of these have been the subject of extensive study, while others quietly do their jobs without attracting a lot of research attention. And when you put them all together – as nature did in bergamot fruit – they combine to significantly help reduce your cholesterol, triglycerides and blood sugar levels.

One rigorously-studied ingredient in bergamot is a super powerful bioflavonoid called naringin, which is responsible for giving the fruit its distinct bitter taste. This natural compound has been put to the test in multiple studies and has come out victorious time and time again...

For example, one study found that naringin on its own was able to lower LDL ('bad') cholesterol by 17 per cent and total cholesterol by 14 per cent in patients suffering from high cholesterol (*Clinical Nutrition. 22(6): 561-568, 2003*).

In addition, two animal studies found that adding naringin to the diets of rats effectively lowered their serum cholesterol levels (*Journal of Nutrition. 129 (6): 1182-1185, 1999; Annals of Nutrition & Metabolism. 45 (5): 193-201, 2001*).

Researchers also found that naringin (along with hesperidin, another natural compound in bergamot) can significantly lower high blood sugar levels – another defining symptom of metabolic syndrome that can lead to full-blown diabetes and its many dangerous complications. One animal study showed that supplementing with this flavonoid substantially lowered blood glucose in mice modelled with type 2 diabetes (*Journal of Nutrition.*

134 (10): 2499-2503, 2004).

Naringin has also been found to be beneficial at lowering high triglyceride levels, which is critical for optimal cardiovascular health.

Metabolic syndrome sufferers lower their triglyceride levels by 49% and blood sugar levels by 22% in just 4 weeks

When it comes to fighting metabolic syndrome, bergamot extract may be your best bet. Because while a single one of its main compounds (naringin) has shown incredible results, its combination of powerful flavonoids really takes the symptoms to task.

In one clinical trial, researchers uncovered the true power of bergamot polyphenolic extract (BPF) (*Mollace, V., et al. Potent hypolipemic and hypoglycemic effect of bergamot-derived poliphenolic fraction: role in 3-hydroxy-3-methyl glutaryl CoA reductase inhibition. (ahead of publication)*). This 30-day, placebo-controlled, interventional study included 238 patients, all of whom had high cholesterol, and some of whom also had high blood sugar levels.

At the end of the 30 days most of the patients in the BPF group had substantially lower total cholesterol levels – up to 38 per cent lower! And their LDL cholesterol levels were just as impressive, with an average 37 per cent drop.

And, according to the researchers, the most impressive changes were seen in a subgroup of patients identified as having metabolic syndrome. Those patients saw a huge dip in their triglyceride levels – up to a 49 per cent drop – and an average 22 per cent drop in blood sugar levels... in just one month.

What to take for best results

While you might not want to suffer through eating the extremely acrid bergamot fruit – even to get results like that – you can get its benefits without taking a single bitter bite. Bergamot polyphenolic extract comes in a unique supplement called Bergamonte.

The manufacturer recommends a therapeutic dose of two to four Bergamonte capsules daily, before dinner, on an empty stomach for the first 30 days. After that, they recommend a maintenance dose of one capsule daily (still before dinner, on an empty stomach).

- **Discover how Body Balance can boost your metabolism, regulate your blood sugar levels and help you lose weight**

If you've considered taking a sports supplement in the past to help you lose weight, gain muscle or retain muscle mass, but been put off by the aisles full of bodybuilding products in your local health food shop, then a new preparation called Body Balance could be just what you're looking for.

Body Balance by Biocare works by combining conjugated linoleic acid (CLA) with L-carnitine, high quality whey protein and chromium, to help promote energy production, fat metabolism and healthy blood sugar levels.

New clinical trials show that CLA aids weight loss with no side effects

A key ingredient in Body Balance is CLA. This is a specific fatty acid found in red meats and dairy products that appears to support the body's management of fats and helps maintain a favourable ratio of lean muscle to fat. CLA helps to block the absorption of fat and sugar into fat cells (adipocytes) and helps the insulin receptors remain intact, so increasing insulin sensitivity. It also has powerful antioxidant and anti-inflammatory activity.

Several animal studies have found that CLA raises metabolic rate and reduces body fat, but until recently the results of human trials have been inconclusive. Now, two new clinical trials have shown that CLA not only aids weight loss and improves body fat composition in humans, but does so without any adverse effects on blood fats or other metabolic indicators.

The first clinical trial was carried out at the Max Rubner Institute in Germany and involved 85 overweight and obese men aged from 45 to 68 years (*J Am Coll Nutr. 2011; 30 (1): 19-28*). It found that CLA reduced body weight as compared to placebo (safflower oil), after four weeks of supplementation. In addition, there were beneficial effects on some measures of oxidative stress and metabolic function, while no adverse changes were seen in blood fat levels or in blood vessel function.

The second study, from China, was a randomized, double-blind, placebo-controlled trial in which 63 overweight people (body mass index 24 to 35) received either CLA or placebo twice a day for 12 weeks (*Nutrition. 2012; 28 (5): 559-565*). In the group receiving CLA, body weight, body mass index, total fat mass, fat percentage, subcutaneous fat mass, and waist-to-hip ratio all decreased, while there were no significant changes in these measurements in the placebo group.

L-carnitine is essential for the fat-burning furnaces in your muscle cells

The amino acid L-carnitine is included in Body Balance because it plays an important role in transporting fatty acids into the mitochondria (energy-producing centres) of cells and in cellular energy release. The oxidation of fatty acids within the mitochondria provides the primary source of energy for the heart and skeletal muscles, underlining the importance of this nutrient for the proper functioning of these tissues.

In theory, healthy adults should be able to make sufficient L-carnitine in their bodies or get enough from their diet, but in fact many people have some degree of carnitine deficiency (*Altern Med Rev. 1998; 3 (5): 345-360*). In rats, age-related decline in the efficiency of the heart muscle has been reversed by supplementation with L-carnitine, according to a new study. L-carnitine appears to work best in assisting weight loss when it is combined with a diet that is low in sugars and starches (carbohydrates) and contains adequate essential fatty acids and protein.

The latter is especially important in terms of promoting weight loss. It is also essential for building muscle and tissue repair. If we don't eat enough protein or get the correct balance of amino acids, then weight loss may prove elusive. The high quality whey protein in Body Balance provides an excellent source of balanced amino acids that the body can use readily.

Researchers recently made an important discovery about the mechanism controlling the body's 'fat switch', shedding new light on our understanding of how proteins regulate appetite control and insulin secretion (*J Biol Chem. 2011; 286 (49): 42545-54*). This involves an enzyme called carnitine palmitoyltransferase 1A, which is involved in the metabolic pathway through which L-carnitine releases energy in the muscle cells. The enzyme plays a critical role in regulating fatty acid oxidation (fat burning) in the body.

Chromium picolinate helps maintain healthy blood sugar levels

Chromium is a trace element that is essential for normal carbohydrate and fat metabolism, and numerous studies have shown that chromium helps to prevent insulin resistance, as well as reducing cholesterol levels (*Mol Cell Biochem. 2008; 317 (1-2): 1-10*). When additional chromium was given to rats fed on a high fat diet, it protected them from becoming obese, according to a study carried out in Turkey in 2011(*Nutr Metab (Lond). 2011; 8:28*).

Human clinical trials have also shown the benefits of chromium. In a randomised, double-blind study at the University of Vermont, in the US, patients with type 2 diabetes were given a chromium picolinate supplement or placebo for six months (*Diabetes Care. 2006; 29 (8): 1826-1832*). Those taking the chromium had better insulin sensitivity and blood sugar control, less weight gain and less visceral fat accumulation than patients in the placebo group.

Chromium is particularly important for people who suffer from diabetes, which often goes hand-in-hand with being overweight or obese. Animal studies have shown that chromium picolinate, as well as preventing the development of type 2 diabetes, also protects against some of its complications, including diabetic nephropathy (kidney damage).

What to take for best results

Body Balance is formulated as a convenient powder that is used to make a pleasant tasting drink. The recommended dose of Body Balance is one scoop (approximately 30g) of powder, mixed in water or milk, taken daily.

Taking regular exercise that includes short bursts of maximum effort, and following a diet that restricts sugar and starches and includes good amounts of protein and omega-3 fatty acids, will help you to lose fat and gain muscle faster.

People who suffer from epilepsy, high blood pressure, or kidney disease, or who are under medical supervision, are advised to talk to their doctor before using Body Balance. It is not suitable for women who are pregnant, planning to become pregnant or breastfeeding.

- **Shed those unwanted pounds once and for all with a brand new slimming aid that also helps stabilise your blood sugar levels**

Numerous studies have revealed a link between coffee consumption and a reduced risk of developing type 2 diabetes. It was previously thought that it was the caffeine in coffee which was responsible for this effect. However, a study of 28,000 women found that drinking more than six cups of decaffeinated coffee a day was associated with a 33 per cent lower risk of diabetes compared with no coffee (*Arch Intern Med. 2006 Jun 26;*

166 (12): 1311-6).

Further research pointed to substances called chlorogenic acids (polyphenols with antioxidant activity) in coffee as being responsible for its beneficial action on glucose metabolism. However, some studies showed that it was necessary to consume copious amounts of coffee for it to have this effect. Consequently this led researchers to develop a coffee bean extract rich in chlorogenic acids which has now been adapted into a natural food supplement.

Derived from decaffeinated Robusta coffee beans (also known as green coffee), the coffee bean extract named Svetol® has been produced to contain specific amounts of different chlorogenic acids. The product also contains caffeic acid, another compound well known for its antioxidant properties. Furthermore, the product is free of caffeine, cafestol and kahweo – compounds which are known to have a detrimental effect on health.

Although Svetol® helps decrease high blood sugar levels after eating, it has also been found to promote weight loss. Studies show that it can significantly reduce body mass index (a measuring tool that allows you to evaluate your body's health status) as well as weight. Its intake has also been reported to reduce sweet cravings and the tendency to snack between meals.

Svetol® helps prevent excess glucose from being turned into fat

When we eat carbohydrate-rich foods such as bread, potatoes, pasta and sugar they are broken down into glucose, which the body uses as an energy source. If there is too much glucose in the blood, some of the excess gets converted into glycogen where it is stored in your liver and the rest into fat where it is stored in the fat depots around your body. Your body can then call upon these glycogen and fat stores when blood sugar levels have dropped below their normal level.

Svetol® works by inhibiting glucose absorption in the intestines, thereby reducing carbohydrate and calorie intake. The result is that your blood sugar 'peak' will be reduced after a meal, and so you have less chance of turning excess glucose into fat.

It has also been found to inhibit the activity of glucose-6-phosphatase – an enzyme responsible for the release of glucose (in the form of glycogen) stored in the liver into general circulation. This means that energy is instead drawn from fat deposits in adipose tissue, which stimulates weight loss.

Study participants taking Svetol® lost 11lbs of weight on average in just 8 weeks

A study undertaken at the Antonio e Margherita Hospital in Tortona, Italy, involving 50 people demonstrated Svetol®'s weight loss action. Over the course of 60 days, two groups of volunteers, all with a body mass index over 25 (this means they were overweight) were observed.

The first group was given 400mg of Svetol® daily, while the second group received a placebo. After 60 days of supplementation, participants who received Svetol® lost 5.7 per cent of their initial weight or an average weight loss of 4.9 kg or 11 lbs. The group that received a placebo lost only 2.8 per cent of their initial weight corresponding to an average of 2.4 kg or 5.2 lbs (*Phytothérapie, November 2006 Volume 4, Number 4*).

In 2005, Dr. Erling Thom from PAREXEL (a company that specialises in managing clinical trials) conducted several trials with Svetol® in Norway. The main study was a randomised, placebo-controlled, double-blind study using Svetol® combined with a calorie-controlled diet over 60 days (*Thom E. The effect of chlorogenic acid (Svetol®) and chlorogenic enriched coffee (CoffeeSlender) on the glucose profile and body weight of healthy volunteers. PAREXEL Medstat AS, Lillestrøm, Norway 2005*). The 30 participants using Svetol® lost more than twice the amount of weight (an average of 5kg or 11lbs) compared to those on the same diet but without Svetol® (an average of 2.4kg or 5.2lbs).

The second study undertaken by Dr. Thom showed that a single dose of Svetol® caused a 20 per cent reduction in glucose levels after one hour compared to eating the same food but without Svetol® (*Thom E. The effect of chlorogenic acid (Svetol®) and chlorogenic enriched coffee (CoffeeSlender) on the glucose profile and body weight of healthy volunteers. PAREXEL Medstat AS, Lillestrøm, Norway 2005*).

The third study was based on a Svetol®-containing coffee beverage called CoffeeSLENDER. Participants were asked not to change their regular diet or exercise habits during the trial. After 90 days the average weight loss was 5.4 kg or 11.8 lbs (*Thom E. The effect of chlorogenic acid (Svetol®) and chlorogenic enriched coffee (CoffeeSlender) on the glucose profile and body weight of healthy volunteers. PAREXEL Medstat AS, Lillestrøm, Norway 2005*).

Another Svetol® study was undertaken in 2002 by Dr James Blum at the University of Maine Department of Food Science and Human Nutrition. In this study, the respondents lost an average of 1.5 kg (more than 3 lbs) in six weeks without diet and exercise changes (*Marshall-Blum, BlumJM and Blum RI. Prospective, nonrandomized, open label non-blinded pilot clinical trial to test the efficiency and short term safety of Svetol® a natural product intended for internal use to lower serum glucose and promote healthy weight loss. University of Maine Department of Food Science and Human Nutrition, Orono, Maine, USA. 2002*).

What to take for best results

Svetol® is available in capsule form in a product called Natessance SLIM (decaffeinated) or as an instant coffee beverage (caffeinated) known as CoffeeSLENDER.

With Natessance SLIM the recommended dosage is one capsule taken with your main meals (with a large glass of water) for a minimum of 50 days. CoffeeSLENDER, which is Svetol® combined with regular caffeinated coffee, should be taken at a dose of two level teaspoons in a cup of hot water after main meals for two months. If you are sensitive to caffeine, it is suggested that only two cups a day are drunk – one after breakfast and one after lunch. Although some of the studies with Svetol® did not involve participants changing their diet, it is advisable to follow a healthy eating plan when taking the supplement, as this will enable weight loss to be sustained.

Contraindications: Svetol® should not be taken during pregnancy or while breastfeeding. Also, people on medication should consult their GP before taking Svetol®-based products.

Svetol® is also a key ingredient in the following supplement by Solgar…

- **This cutting-edge new supplement helps burn fat, boosts energy, and keeps blood sugar levels stable**

If you're trying to lose weight then a cutting-edge new supplement called Thermogenic Complex with Svetol® by Solgar could provide the solution. The formula combines eight key ingredients – Svetol® green coffee, green tea, cayenne pepper, black pepper extract and chromium, along with choline, inositol and methionine – that work together to help kick-start your metabolism and promote weight loss.

Thermogenic Complex with Svetol®, as its name suggests, increases thermogenesis – the body's process of burning fat in the production of heat. Thermogenesis stimulates your basal metabolic rate (BMR) – the amount of energy needed to maintain your body's basic functions at a cellular level – which tends to slow down with age.

As well as boosting your energy levels and helping your body burn fat, the formula's thermogenic action also promotes overall good health as it plays an integral role in utilising nutrients from the food we eat – setting in motion the mechanisms that lead to optimal digestion and subsequent gastrointestinal absorption.

The incredible weight-loss and fat burning capabilities of Svetol® green coffee, green tea and capsaicin

As mentioned earlier, Svetol® green coffee is the term used to refer to the unprocessed coffee bean. The normal roasting process, designed to release the aroma and flavour of coffee, destroys some of its active components, including chlorogenic acid. It is chlorogenic acid that can reduce blood glucose levels and promote fat loss. Its ability to increase lean body mass has been the subject of several studies.

One study lasting 22 weeks examined the efficacy and safety of green coffee extract in reducing weight and body mass in 16 overweight adults (*Diabetes Metab Syndr Obes 2012; 5: 21-7. Epub 2012 Jan 18*). Those taking part in the study had three separate six-week treatment periods, separated by two-week rest periods. In one period they received high doses of green coffee extract, in another low doses of the same extract, and in the third only a placebo.

Significant reductions were observed in body weight, body mass index and the percentage of body fat, and there was also a small decrease in heart rate, when the subjects took green coffee extract. And in six cases the weight loss was enough to shift them from being defined as 'pre-obese' to 'normal weight'. The researchers concluded that green coffee extract could be effective in reducing weight in 'pre-obese' adults, and an inexpensive means of preventing obesity in overweight adults.

A recent review of studies has revealed that green tea – another key ingredient in Thermogenic Complex with Svetol® – can promote weight loss (*Br J Nutr. 2011 Nov; 106 (9): 1297-309. Epub 2011 Aug 3*). It contains a small amount of caffeine, which serves as a mild appetite suppressant. In addition, studies suggest that green tea extracts high in catechins are able to activate fat-burning mechanisms in the body and increase the conversion from fat to energy (*Am J Clin Nutr 1999 70, 1040-45; Nutrition Research, Volume 26, Issue 11, November 2006, Pages 604-607*).

Studies indicate that it is this combination of caffeine and catechins, which makes green tea so effective at combating obesity (*In Vivo 2004 18, 55-62; Int J Obes Relat Metab Disord 2000 24, 252-58*). Researchers have also found that it can help ward off metabolic syndrome as a result of its ability to slow down the absorption of fat after meals and by reducing the deposit of 'visceral fat' around the organs in the abdomen (*Asia Pac J Clin Nutr 2008; 17 (Suppl) 1: 273-274*).

Cayenne pepper has been included in the formula as it contains capsaicin, which stimulates lipolysis – the breakdown of stored body fat for energy use (*Phytother Res 2011 Jun; 25(6): 935-9. doi: 10.1002/ptr.3339. Epub 2010 Nov 17*). It helps reduce appetite, speeds up metabolism, inhibits fat cell growth and prevents fat cell formation. An animal study revealed that capsaicin reduces weight gain and white adipose (fat) tissue formation in rats (*Journal of Proteome Research, June 2010*).

Other research has shown the benefits of both capsaicin and green tea in suppressing hunger and increasing the feeling of satiety (*Clin Nutr. 2009 Jun; 28 (3): 260-5. Epub 2009 Apr 3*).

The remaining ingredients in the formula also help shift excess weight

Black pepper (thanks to its key ingredient, piperine) enhances the body's natural thermogenic – fat burning – activity. Not only does it 'power up' the process of thermogenesis, but it also helps the body make more efficient use of nutrients. Solgar's Thermogenic Complex with Svetol® contains a black pepper extract that has been patented for its ability to increase the bioavailability of nutritional compounds.

Thermogenic Complex with Svetol® also contains chromium – a trace element that is essential for normal carbohydrate and fat metabolism. One study assessed the effects of chromium in a group of 42 overweight women who said they craved carbohydrates (*Anton SD, Morrison CD, Cefalu WT, Martin CK, Coulon S, Geiselman P, Han H, White CL, Williamson DA. Effects of chromium picolinate on food intake and satiety. Pennington Biomedical Research Center, Louisiana State University, Baton Rouge, Louisiana, USA).*

This double-blind, placebo-controlled study randomly assigned the women to receive doses of chromium or a placebo for eight weeks. The researchers found that chromium reduced food intake, hunger levels and cravings, and also encouraged weight loss. Research has also revealed that chromium can enhance the metabolic action of insulin and appears to have a blood sugar lowering effect.

The remaining three ingredients – choline (an essential nutrient), inositol (a carbohydrate produced from glucose) and methionine (an essential amino acid) – are all 'lipotropic' agents, meaning that they help to break down fat in the body. Ideally they should be obtained from our diet, but deficiencies can occur and cause subsequent problems. For example, a deficiency of choline and inositol impedes the breakdown of fat. Methionine and choline also help to detoxify waste generated by the breakdown of proteins in the body.

What to take for best results

The recommended dosage for Thermogenic Complex with Svetol® is two capsules per day. As previously mentioned, Svetol® should not be taken during pregnancy or while breastfeeding. Also, people on medication should consult their GP before taking Svetol®-based products.

For best results, the supplement should be taken in conjunction with regular exercise and a low GL diet, which eliminates processed foods and refined carbohydrates.

• **Discover the plant extract that is proving successful in the fight against diabetes**

Elecampane (*Inula helenium*) is a perennial plant that grows throughout Europe and Asia and produces distinct yellow spiky flowers... which is how it gained its nickname 'wild sunflower.'

It has been used in folk medicine for thousands of years and was prized by ancient Greek healers as an effective remedy for the treatment of respiratory problems like coughs, bronchitis and emphysema.

It is still used for this purpose today and also as a beneficial treatment for numerous other disorders including diabetes, circulation problems, joint pains and indigestion. It is also an effective tonic that promotes overall well-being.

Promising news for managing diabetes

Elecampane root is a rich source of inulin – a carbohydrate-based fibre, which helps regulate blood sugar levels.

In an animal study, scientists from the Thyroid Research Unit, School of Life Sciences, Indore, in India, looked at the effect the root extract has on blood sugar levels. They studied the effect of the plant on its own and, at a later stage, in association with another anti-diabetic herb called gymnema sylvestre. They found that both plants were able to significantly lower blood sugar levels when taken individually but were far more effective when given in combination (*Eksp Klin Farmakol. 2003 Jul-Aug; 66 (4): 63-5*).

The root extract has also been found to prevent another detrimental effect caused by too much sugar. Scientists have discovered that it helps protect against a process called glycosylation – chemical damage to your cells and proteins caused by excess sugar – which can stress internal organs like your heart and liver (*Gholap S, Kar A. Pharmazie. 2003 Jun; 58 (6): 413-5*).

Root extract helps defend against harmful free radicals

Japanese scientists from the Faculty of Pharmaceutical Sciences, at the University of Tokushima, examined several Asian herbs, including

Elecampane, for their ability to reduce levels of harmful free radicals such as nitric oxide and oxygen peroxide.

Free radicals are dangerous chemicals that are implicated in causing numerous serious conditions, including cancer, and are produced by your cells following exposure to pollution, cigarette smoke, alcohol and stress.

When the scientists studied Elecampane they discovered that it contains several hitherto unknown about chemicals – variants of sesquiterpene lactones – that have turned out to be powerful antioxidants that can neutralise harmful free radicals (*Phytomedicine. 2004 Nov; 11(7-8): 645-51*).

What to take for best results

The recommended dosage for Elecampane root is two capsules (each containing 503mg of Elecampane root) taken three times a day with water – or as otherwise directed on the product's label.

For the treatment of diabetes, Elecampane can be more effective when taken alongside gymnema sylvestre – the recommended dosage for this herb is one 300mg capsule a day. It is important that you consult your doctor first before taking either herb, especially if you are currently on any medication.

Contraindications: Pregnant and breast-feeding women should not use Elecampane.

- **Aronia – This antioxidant powerhouse helps fight everything from cancer to metabolic syndrome**

Antioxidants are extremely important for maintaining good health. In particular they help to reverse the harmful effects of oxidative stress, which is implicated in numerous chronic diseases including cancer (*Med Oncol 2005; 22 (1): 11-15*).

Oxidative stress involves cellular damage caused by free radicals – reactive molecules that are by-products of normal and essential metabolic processes that take place every day in your body; they are also produced as a result of stress, pollution, smoking and poor diet.

Some of the most potent antioxidants are plant chemicals called polyphenols, found in a wide range of fruits and vegetables as well as in green tea, chocolate, red wine and olive oil. A lot of the research on polyphenols has focused on a sub-group called flavonoids, which have been linked to numerous health benefits, due to their ability to protect cell structures and membranes and to reduce inflammation. In some cases, flavonoids can also act directly as antibiotics, helping to fight viruses and bacteria.

Plants are thought to produce flavonoids to protect them against the free radicals generated by exposure to sunshine, and they have a similar antioxidant effect in the body. They trigger the production of natural enzymes and powerful disease-fighting antioxidants like glutathione in the body (*Free Radic Biol Med 2006; 41(12): 1727-1746*).

Flavonoids have been found to help reduce the risk of certain cancers, heart disease, and age-related degenerative illnesses. Research also indicates that they may help prevent skin ageing, macular degeneration and tooth decay, and reduce the occurrence of common ailments such as influenza.

Berries are one of the best natural sources of flavonoids, with blueberries, blackberries, raspberries and cranberries all showing disease-fighting properties (*Mol Nutr Food Res 2007; 51(6): 675-83*). But, in recent years, one berry has been found to have antioxidant properties way above all the rest: Aronia.

Although aronia berries are jam packed full of beneficial flavonoids, their flavour is so sour that they are almost impossible to eat raw, or to take as unsweetened juice. Fortunately, aronia is now available in the UK in supplement form, from the German company Pascoe Naturmedizin, as

ARONIA-PASCOE® capsules.

This incredible berry tops the antioxidant league

Aronia is also known as the chokeberry – not to be confused with the chokecherry, a completely different plant that helps fight cold and flu viruses. Aronia is a dark purple berry that is native to North America but is more popular nowadays in Russia and Eastern Europe, where its juice is drunk regularly for its health-giving properties.

When the US Department of Agriculture tested the antioxidant capacity of a huge range of foods in 2007, aronia topped all other fresh fruits and vegetables (*Oxygen radical absorbance capacity (ORAC) of selected foods. Nutrient Data Laboratory, Agriculture Research Service, US Department of Agriculture, 2007*). Its 'oxygen radical absorbance capacity' (ORAC) value – a standard measure of antioxidant capacity – was 16,062, compared with 14,697 for elderberry, 9,584 for cranberry and 6,552 for blueberry.

The evidence for aronia's disease-fighting powers is strong. A research review published in April 2010 confirmed that not only is it a very powerful antioxidant but that it may also specifically prevent diabetes, cell mutations and cancers, protect the heart, liver and digestive system, fight bacteria and viruses and support the immune system, while suppressing inflammation (*J Med Food 2010; 13 (2): 255-269*).

Aronia reduces blood sugar, blood pressure and cholesterol levels

In a recent clinical trial carried out at the Medical University of Lodz, Poland, 25 people with metabolic syndrome were given aronia extract for two months (*Med Sci Monit 2010; 16 (1): CR28-34*). Blood tests were carried out before and at the end of the study.

The results were dramatic. Average systolic blood pressure dropped 12 points, from 143 to 131 mmHg, while levels of low density lipoprotein ('bad' cholesterol) and blood sugar also fell significantly.

At the same time, there were marked increases in the amounts of circulating antioxidant enzymes – for instance, there was a more than 50 per cent rise in glutathione peroxidise, which is one of the body's main antioxidant enzymes and has been found to protect against DNA damage, toxins and carcinogens, enhance immune function and prevent the oxidation of cholesterol (it is the oxidised kind that causes cardiovascular disease).

What to take for best results

The recommended dosage is two ARONIA-PASCOE® capsules taken twice daily, either before or after meals. The capsules should be swallowed whole with water.

A final word of advice

Your best strategy for avoiding or managing type 1 or type 2 diabetes is to take control... and after reading *Diabetes Defeated: 97 Most Powerful Secrets For Controlling Blood Sugar Levels Naturally* you now have all the information at hand to successfully manage your blood sugar levels.

The importance of making simple lifestyle changes can't be emphasised enough. Following the right diet, in addition to taking regular exercise, getting enough sleep, and maintaining a healthy weight, is crucial for regulating blood sugar levels – remember, in its early stages type 2 diabetes is fully reversible.

A low GL diet is the key to achieving this... as is cutting sugar out of your diet as much as possible. This approach, combined with the latest cutting-edge natural breakthroughs and safe alternatives outlined in this report can help bring your blood sugar levels down and help minimise your reliance on drugs.

Although medications have their place in the treatment of diabetes and are sometimes essential, you should work with your doctor to reduce your need for them as they all have side effects, some of which are life-threatening. The measures outlined in *Diabetes Defeated: 97 Most Powerful Secrets For Controlling Blood Sugar Levels Naturally* should help with this.

As emphasised throughout *Diabetes Defeated: 97 Most Powerful Secrets For Controlling Blood Sugar Levels Naturally* it's important to bear in mind that every person's diabetes is different and you should work closely with your doctor. It's also extremely important that you discuss any changes you plan to make with your doctor and you should never stop taking any medication without consulting your doctor first.

In addition to regularly monitoring your own blood sugar levels and making sure your doctor regularly monitors them too, it's vital that you demand to have all the necessary checks carried out in order to avoid

239

diabetes-related complications. Don't assume that doctors and nurses know best, or even know what they are doing... recent reports highlighting the poor levels of diabetes care in the UK are testament to that.

Following the advice in *Diabetes Defeated: 97 Most Powerful Secrets For Controlling Blood Sugar Levels Naturally* will not only help stabilise your blood sugar levels and transform your health (your risk of cardiovascular disease will be dramatically reduced for starters), your waistline and energy levels will also benefit enormously.

Further reading

The GL Diet Recipe Book and Health Plan: Everything You Need to Know About the Glycaemic Loading Approach to Weight Loss and Good Health by Maggie Pannell. A concise, but very comprehensive, explanation of GI (Glycaemic Index) and GL (Glycaemic Load) principles, plus a large selection of recipes, illustrated with full colour photographs. It's not aimed specifically at people with diabetes, but explains clearly how low GI/GL foods promote stable blood sugar control, in addition to numerous other health benefits.

Say No To Diabetes: 10 Healthy Ways to Prevent or Reverse Diabetes by Patrick Holford. Nutrition expert Patrick Holford provides an anti-diabetes diet, recipes, a daily supplement programme and advice on how to undo the damage caused by diabetes and diabetes drugs. Based on the latest scientific findings, combined with easy-to-follow advice and motivating case histories, this practical programme will help you regulate out-of-control blood sugar levels safely and effectively, with no dangerous side effects.

Sugar Nation: The Hidden Truth Behind America's Deadliest Habit and the Simple Way to Beat It by Jeff O' Connell. Reveals the true dangers of sugar and how it is a large contributing factor to diabetes and many other diseases. It also explores diabetes – from diagnosis and treatment, to the failings of modern medical science in treating patients effectively. Told by a young man who was diagnosed as pre-diabetic shortly after his estranged father lost his life to diabetic complications (including amputation) – this is his journey in finding an effective way to keep his blood sugar levels even, to prevent and treat diabetes by way of diet and lifestyle modification, not medicine.

Atkins Diabetes Revolution: Control Your Carbs to Prevent and Manage Type 2 Diabetes (Based on the Medical Practice of Dr. Robert C. Atkins) by Dr. Mary C. Vernon (a GP on the Atkins Physicians Council) and Jacqueline A. Eberstein R.N. (a nurse who worked with Dr. Atkins for almost 20 years and is now on the staff of Atkins Health & Medical Information Services). The Atkins organisation is renowned for their work on diabetes and this book sets out a controlled carb diet and nutrition regime to help people lose weight and prevent, treat and even reverse diabetes. The Atkins nutritional plan, based on eating the foods that balance your hormones to regulate blood sugar levels, controls the production of insulin and is therefore a great tool in treating and preventing diabetes. The Atkins plan also promotes healthy weight loss and freedom from other conditions, such as high blood pressure and heart disease.

Dr. Bernstein's Diabetes Solution: A Complete Guide To Achieving Normal Blood Sugars, 3rd Edition, by Dr. Richard Bernstein. Since its first publication in 1997 *Diabetes Solution* has become the treatment of choice in the medical field in America. Dr. Bernstein's ground-breaking approach to diabetes care enables patients to take control of their disease to live long and healthy lives by regulating their blood sugar without the usual swings. Dr. Bernstein is living proof of the success of his method and in this revised and updated edition of his work he gives an accessible, detailed guide to his revolutionary approach and outlines his plan for preventing or reversing long-term complications of the disease. He offers the most up-to-date information on new products, medications and supplements and explains the connection between obesity and age-onset diabetes. In this revised edition, he adds 40 new gourmet, low carbohydrate recipes in addition to the original 50.

There Is a Cure for Diabetes: The Tree of Life 21-day+ Program by Gabriel Cousens. Dr. Cousens' method, widely tested at his famous Tree of Life centres, is to reset the DNA through green juice fasting and a 100% organic, nutrient-dense, vegan, low-glycaemic, low-insulin-scoring, and high-mineral diet of living foods in the first twenty-one days. Both practical and inspirational, the book explains how to abandon the widespread "culture of death"– symbolized by addictive junk food – that fosters diabetes in favour of a more natural, nurturing approach. The program claims to render insulin and related medicines unnecessary within four days as the blood sugar drops to normal levels; and the diabetic shifts into a non-diabetic physiology within two weeks. The third week focuses on live-food preparation, featuring 100 delicious raw recipes. Dr. Cousens emphasizes regular consultations, monitoring blood chemistries, and emotional support, and includes a one-year support program to help maintain a diabetes-free life.

Managing Your Gestational Diabetes: A Guide for You and Your Baby's Good Health by Lois Jovanovic-Peterson. An informative guide to gestational diabetes and how to control it, in order to minimise the risks for both you and your child.

Helpful organisations

Diabetes UK. Leading UK diabetes charity that helps people with diabetes and their families. They provide information, advice and support and also fund research into the condition. Careline: 0845 120 2960 (Monday–Friday, 9am–5pm); Website: www.diabetes.org.uk

Diabetes.co.uk provides information on type 1 and type 2 diabetes. There is also an online forum where sufferers can contact other sufferers. Website: www.diabetes.co.uk

Juvenile Diabetes Research Foundation (JDRF). A charity for sufferers of type 1 diabetes. They fund research to cure, treat and prevent type 1 diabetes, and provide information for children, adults and parents living with the condition, at all stages from diagnosis and beyond. Tel: 020 7713 2030; Website: www.jdrf.org.uk

Insulindependence. Helps empower diabetes sufferers. Teaches sufferers how to effectively manage their condition through exercise and active living. Website: www.insulindependence.org

The Real Diabetes Truth. Nutritional therapist Martin Hum (PhD DHD) provides expert advice in this dedicated diabetes blog and brings you news on the very latest cutting-edge natural breakthroughs and safe alternatives that can help bring your blood sugar levels down and transform your health. Visit: www.realdiabetestruth.com

NHS Choices. Provides healthcare advice and information, including a section on diabetes. Website: www.nhschoices.nhs.uk

NHS 24. Confidential telephone health advice and information service for people in Scotland. Tel: 08454 242424; Website: www.nhs24.com

The Diabetes Research Institute. The largest and most comprehensive diabetes research centre dedicated to curing diabetes.
Website: www.diabetesresearch.org

European Association for the Study of Diabetic Eye Complications.
Information and advice on all the eye complications that diabetes may cause.
Website: http://medweb.bham.ac.uk/easdec/index.html

Moorfields Eye Hospital: retinal disease. This site covers most eye illnesses and conditions, including those caused by diabetes. Helpline: 020 7566 2345; Website: www.moorfields.nhs.uk

UK National Kidney Federation. Run by kidney patients for kidney patients. Promotes the welfare of people with kidney disease or renal failure, and the relatives and friends who care for them. Helpline: 0845 601 0209; Website: www.kidney.org.uk

The Pituitary Foundation: diabetes insipidus. Provides information and support to people with pituitary disorders, of which diabetes insipidus is one. Tel: 0845 450 0376; Website: www.pituitary.org.uk

The Society of Chiropodists and Podiatrists. Provides information on how to prevent and treat common foot problems, including those caused by diabetes. Website: www.feetforlife.org

The British Association for Counselling and Psychotherapy. BACP House, 15 St John's Business Park, Lutterworth, Leics LE17 4HB. Tel: 01455 883300; Website: www.bacp.co.uk

Institute for Complementary and Natural Medicine. Supplies contact details of practitioners of various kinds of complementary medicine. Tel: 0207 922 7980; Website: www.icnm.org.uk

The British Association for Nutritional Therapy, 27 Old Gloucester Street, London WC1N 3XX. Tel: 0870 606 1284; Website: www.bant.org.uk

The Green People (www.greenpeople.co.uk) manufacture a range of skin care, hair care and cosmetic products that don't use any harsh chemicals and select only the finest natural and organic ingredients. In addition they use fair trade ingredients that have not been tested on animals. They also produce chemical-free products for babies.

The Nutri Centre. The UK's leading supplier of vitamin and mineral supplements and herbal remedies. Tel: 0207 436 5122; Website: www.nutricentre.com

Revital. Online health store that supplies a wide range of nutritional supplements, health foods and herbal remedies. Tel: 0800 252 875; Website: www.revital.co.uk

DATE DUE